New Updates in Oral and Maxillofacial Surgery

New Updates in Oral and Maxillofacial Surgery

Guest Editors

Fabio Maglitto
Giovanni Salzano

MDPI
Basel • Beijing • Wuhan • Barcelona • Belgrade • Novi Sad • Cluj • Manchester

Guest Editors
Fabio Maglitto
Maxillofacial Surgery Unit, Department of Interdisciplinary Medicine
Aldo Moro University of Bari
Bari
Italy

Giovanni Salzano
Department of Reproductive and Odontostomatological Neurosciences
University of Naples "Federico II"
Naples
Italy

Editorial Office
MDPI AG
Grosspeteranlage 5
4052 Basel, Switzerland

This is a reprint of the Special Issue, published open access by the journal *Journal of Personalized Medicine* (ISSN 2075-4426), freely accessible at: https://www.mdpi.com/journal/jpm/special_issues/W9949PQRH7.

For citation purposes, cite each article independently as indicated on the article page online and as indicated below:

Lastname, A.A.; Lastname, B.B. Article Title. *Journal Name* **Year**, *Volume Number*, Page Range.

ISBN 978-3-7258-5771-5 (Hbk)
ISBN 978-3-7258-5772-2 (PDF)
https://doi.org/10.3390/books978-3-7258-5772-2

Contents

Journal of *Personalized Medicine*

MDPI

Editorial

Special Issue "New Updates in Oral and Maxillofacial Surgery"

Fabio Maglitto [1,*], Chiara Copelli [1], Alfonso Manfuso [1], Stefan Cocis [1] and Giovanni Salzano [2]

1 Maxillo-Facial Surgery, Interdisciplinary Department of Medicine, University of Bari, 70100 Bari, Italy; chiara.copelli@uniba.it (C.C.); alfonso.manfuso@policlinic.ba.it (A.M.); stefan.cocis@policlinico.ba.it (S.C.)

2 Maxillofacial Surgery Unit, Department of Neurosciences, Reproductive and Odontostomatological Sciences, University of Naples Federico II, 80131 Naples, Italy; giovannisalzanomd@gmail.com

* Correspondence: fabio.maglitto@policlinico.ba.it; Tel.: +39-0805593124; Fax: +39-0805593124

1. Introduction

In the ever-evolving landscape of medical science, few fields have witnessed as profound a transformation as oral and maxillofacial surgery. With each passing year, the integration of cutting-edge technology, innovative techniques, and personalized approaches is redefining the boundaries of what is possible in the realm of maxillofacial and head and neck reconstruction. The advent of digital imaging, precision planning, and minimally invasive procedures has ushered in a new era of patient-centered care and enhanced treatment outcomes.

The Special Issue titled "New Updates in Oral and Maxillofacial Surgery" serves as a guide to the dynamic nature of this discipline. By delving into the latest developments and future trends, it encapsulates the spirit of progress that defines oral and maxillofacial surgery today.

At the forefront of this paradigm shift is the emphasis on personalized treatment modalities. From digital impressions to intricate sterolithographic modeling, the ability to tailor interventions to the unique anatomical and physiological characteristics of each patient has become paramount. This personalized approach not only enhances precision, but also minimizes the risk of complications, ensuring optimal results and patient satisfaction.

The advent of AI can completely change the paradigms of medicine. Chat-Based Generative Pre-trained Transformer (ChatGPT) is an advanced artificial intelligence (AI) language model developed by Open Artificial Intelligence. With regard to head and neck disciplines, Vaira et al. [1] demonstrated AI's ability to resolve complex clinical scenarios, but it still falls short of being considered a reliable support for the decision-making process of specialists in head–neck surgery.

Central to the digital revolution is the emergence of digital impressions and 3D modeling. Traditionally, the process of obtaining dental impressions was laborious and uncomfortable for patients. However, with the advent of intraoral scanners [2], we now offer our patients a more comfortable and efficient alternative. These digital impressions not only streamline the treatment process, but also enable us to achieve unprecedented accuracy in the fabrication of prosthetic restorations and orthognathic surgical planning.

Moreover, 3D planning has emerged as a cornerstone of contemporary oral and maxillofacial surgery. Through sophisticated software algorithms and computer-aided design (CAD) technologies [3–5], we can meticulously plan complex procedures, such as orthognathic surgery and implant placement, with precision and predictability. This level of preoperative planning not only optimizes surgical outcomes, but also minimizes intraoperative complications and reduces patient morbidity.

As discussed by Tian et al. [6] in their review, 3D printing is often used for digital imaging in surgical planning, custom surgical devices, and patient–physician communication.

In parallel, minimally invasive surgery has gained prominence as a preferred approach in the management of craniofacial pathologies. Endoscopic and functional surgery techniques have revolutionized our ability to access and treat complex anatomical regions with minimal disruption to surrounding tissues. These approaches not only result in faster recovery times and reduced postoperative pain, but also preserve aesthetic and functional outcomes for our patients. As demonstrated by Bartholomew et al. [7], the combinations between 3D endoscopy and surgical navigation has the potential to improve surgical efficiency, economy of motion, and safety for the patient.

As we navigate the landscape of oral and maxillofacial surgery, we remain steadfast in our commitment to addressing a diverse array of pathologies, including head and neck surgery, oral cancer, and reconstructive surgery. Augmented reality represents the most innovative approach to translate virtual planning for real patients, as it merges the digital world with the surgical field in real time. Surgeons can access patient-specific data directly within their field of view, through dedicated visors. In head and neck surgical oncology, augmented reality systems overlay critical anatomical information onto the surgeon's visual field [8,9].

In particular, the management of oral cancer poses a significant clinical challenge, demanding a multidisciplinary approach and innovative diagnostic and therapeutic strategies [10,11]. Through collaborative efforts and cutting-edge research, we strive to improve early detection, enhance treatment efficacy, and optimize long-term outcomes for patients afflicted by this devastating disease.

Furthermore, reconstructive surgery continues to play a pivotal role in restoring form and function following trauma, congenital anomalies, or oncologic resections. As discussed by Garajei et al., the virtual surgical planning technique resulted in better facial symmetry and superior esthetic outcomes compared with the conventional technique [12]. Advances in biomaterials, tissue engineering, and microsurgical techniques have expanded the repertoire of reconstructive options available to us, enabling us to achieve remarkable outcomes and improve quality of life for our patients.

2. An Overview of Published Articles

In Andreas Sakkas's paper [13], the author explores the prevalence of challenging airway situations and urgent tracheostomy procedures in individuals with orofacial infections arising from the mandible, as well as methods for identifying factors that may predict difficult intubation. The frequency of challenging airway situations related to breathing, visualizing the larynx, and inserting a breathing tube was studied using descriptive methods. The relationships between possible factors that could affect difficult intubation were investigated through multivariable analysis. The highest occurrence of challenging intubation occurred in patients with infections in the masseteric–mandibular space (42.6%), then in infections of the floor of the mouth (40%), and, finally, in infections in the pterygomandibular space (23.5%). Breathing difficulties and noisy breathing were not linked to the site of infection. The researchers concluded that there was a high prevalence of difficult airway situations in patients with orofacial infections originating in the mandible. Advanced age, restricted mouth opening, a higher Mallampati classification, and a higher Cormack–Lehane grade were identified as dependable indicators of challenging intubation.

The study conducted by Gonzalez-Perez and colleagues [14] examines the use of total joint replacement for immediate reconstruction following ablative surgery for primary tumors affecting the temporo-mandibular joint. In their case series, the researchers emphasized the effectiveness of surgically placing TMJ prostheses in significantly reducing pain levels and TMJ dysfunction resulting from tumor-related TMJ pathology. This retrospective analysis primarily targeted cases where the TMJ was extensively damaged due to various tumors. Compared to alternative reconstructive procedures like costochondral or sternoclavicular grafts, utilizing a TMJ prosthesis can shorten surgery duration and hospital stay while offering immediate functionality without donor site morbidity. TMJ replacement is typically viewed as a final option in the surgical management of TMJ disorder and is considered the preferred approach for immediate reconstruction post-ablative surgery for primary TMJ tumors.

The third article by Boschetti et al. [15] examines the effectiveness of using fat grafts in parotidectomy surgeries. The patients in the study all underwent partial or complete parotidectomy with autologous en bloc dermal fat graft reconstruction. Pre- and post-operative contrast-enhanced MRI scans were performed on all patients. Positive feedback from patients on the cosmetic results, along with validation from the radiology team, supports fat grafting as a successful and safe surgical procedure, even in cases with malignant lesions. The authors conclude that fat grafting is highly successful in terms of aesthetics, procedure duration, and safety during oncological follow-up, consolidating the role of a key technique in craniofacial reconstructive surgery.

The fourth article in this Special Issue, authored by Ho et al. [16], presents a preliminary examination of the impact of surgical precision in maxillomandibular advancement (MMA) on obstructive sleep apnea (OSA) patients. The study specifically looks at how advancements in the maxilla and mandible, as well as counter-clockwise rotation, relate to the reduction in the relative apnea hypopnea index (AHI). This research highlights the significance of recognizing surgical inaccuracies in MMA procedures for OSA patients and emphasizes the importance of increased awareness among surgeons and future research efforts.

The article by Antunez-Conde Hidalgo [17] compared the conventional technique and the customized guided surgery for genioplasty. Genioplasty is a common surgical procedure in the field of maxillofacial surgery. Improvements in facial reconstructive surgery have led to lower risk and more consistent outcomes. This study compares traditional genioplasty with a new surgical technique based on virtual surgical planning, CAD-CAM cutting guides, and custom-made plates for patients.

Serree and colleagues [18] conducted a study to evaluate the precision of a novel MD (PirifixTM) for assisting surgeons in positioning the upper dental arch (UDA) during Le Fort I osteotomies (LFIOs). The PirifixTM, developed by Ennoïa in Besançon, France, is a bone-supported device designed to conform to the lower part of the piriform orifice's anatomy. It serves as an alternative to existing methods for UDA positioning in LFIO procedures. This initial investigation was performed on a 3D-printed model without soft tissue to demonstrate the efficacy of the PirifixTM. However, further research, incorporating facial soft tissue and input from other surgeons, is necessary to validate its effectiveness. PirifixTM could potentially have a significant impact on the performance of complex movements that involve multiple rotations and translations. Further investigation into the use of PirifixTM for complex movements is warranted to fully understand its potential benefits and applications.

Lee's research [19] delves into the nasal dimension using Cone-Beam Computed Tomography. The morphology of the nasal cavity is crucial not only in clinical settings, but also in forensic science. However, previous studies have mainly focused on comparing sexes, so it is important to explore how nasal dimensions correspond to facial and nose dimensions. The authors want to determine whether nasal cavity size varies based on sex, facial index (FI), and nasal index (NI). Lee and colleagues examined CBCT data from 100 patients at Dankook University's dental hospital. Their results indicated that nasal cavity sizes did indeed differ according to sex, FI, and NI. These findings have implications for personalized surgeries in clinical practice and future studies on nasal cavity anatomy.

In their study, Onica et al. [20] share their clinical findings regarding a subperiosteal jaw implant as an alternative for patients with insufficient bone height, who cannot undergo traditional endosseous implants without extensive bone grafting or augmentation procedures. The success of these implants largely depends on the biotype of the gingiva, which influences the quality and quantity of the surrounding soft tissues. The objective of this research is to discuss a newly designed subperiosteal jaw implant through their 6-year clinical experience.

The findings reveal that subperiosteal implant-supported hybrid prostheses, created using digital planning and guided surgery, have yielded disappointing outcomes with only a 25% success rate after 6 years.

3. Conclusions

This collection of articles dedicated to the new updates in oral and maxillofacial surgery demonstrate the richness of the research field. Ranging from retrospective studies to case series and technical notes, several study methods have been used to analyze the use of new technologies in our field of interest.

Our Special Issue provides a platform to explore the latest advancements and future trends in these critical areas of our specialty.

In conclusion, the field of oral and maxillofacial surgery stands at the cusp of a new era—an era defined by digitalization, personalized care, and innovation.

This Special Issue serves as a guide to the ingenuity and dedication of the global maxillofacial surgery community, as we strive to push the boundaries of knowledge and redefine the standards of patient care. As we embark on this journey of discovery and advancement, let us remain steadfast in our commitment to excellence and compassion, guided by the principle of putting our patients' needs first. Together, we will continue to shape the future of oral and maxillofacial surgery, ensuring brighter tomorrows for generations to come.

Author Contributions: Conceptualization, F.M. and G.S.; methodology, C.C.; investigation, A.M. and S.C.; writing—original draft preparation, A.M.; writing—review and editing, F.M., C.C. and G.S. All authors have read and agreed to the published version of the manuscript.

Funding: This research received no external funding.

Conflicts of Interest: The authors declare no conflicts of interest.

References

1. Vaira, L.A.; Lechien, J.R.; Abbate, V.; Allevi, F.; Audino, G.; Beltramini, G.A.; Bergonzani, M.; Bolzoni, A.; Committeri, U.; Crimi, S.; et al. Accuracy of ChatGPT-Generated Information on Head and Neck and Oromaxillofacial Surgery: A Multicenter Collaborative Analysis. *Otolaryngol. Head Neck Surg.* **2023**, *170*, 1492–1503. [CrossRef] [PubMed]
2. Esposito, R.; Masedu, F.; Cicciù, M.; Tepedino, M.; Denaro, M.; Ciavarella, D. Reliabilty of recording occlusal contacts by using intraoral scanner and articulating paper—A prospective study. *J. Dent.* **2024**, *142*, 104872. [CrossRef] [PubMed]
3. Maglitto, F.; Orabona, G.D.; Committeri, U.; Salzano, G.; De Fazio, G.R.; Vaira, L.A.; Abbate, V.; Bonavolontà, P.; Piombino, P.; Califano, L. Virtual Surgical Planning and the "In-House" Rapid Prototyping Technique in Maxillofacial Surgery: The Current Situation and Future Perspectives. *Appl. Sci.* **2021**, *11*, 1009. [CrossRef]
4. Cocozza, S.; Russo, C.; Pontillo, G.; Ugga, L.; Macera, A.; Cervo, A.; De Liso, M.; Di Paolo, N.; Ginocchio, M.I.; Giordano, F.; et al. Is advanced neuroimaging for neuroradiologists? A systematic review of the scientific literature of the last decade. *Neuroradiology* **2016**, *58*, 1233–1239. [CrossRef] [PubMed]
5. Jones, E.A.; Huang, A.T. Virtual Surgical Planning in Head and Neck Reconstruction. *Otolaryngol. Clin. N. Am.* **2023**, *56*, 813–822. [CrossRef] [PubMed]
6. Tian, Y.; Chen, C.; Xu, X.; Wang, J.; Hou, X.; Li, K.; Lu, X.; Shi, H.; Lee, E.S.; Jiang, H.B. A Review of 3D Printing in Dentistry: Technologies, Affecting Factors, and Applications. *Scanning* **2021**, *2021*, 9950131. [CrossRef] [PubMed]
7. Bartholomew, R.A.; Zhou, H.; Boreel, M.; Suresh, K.; Gupta, S.; Mitchell, M.B.; Hong, C.; Lee, S.E.; Smith, T.R.; Guenette, J.P.; et al. Surgical Navigation in the Anterior Skull Base Using 3-Dimensional Endoscopy and Surface Reconstruction. *JAMA Otolaryngol. Head Neck Surg.* **2024**, *150*, 318–326. [CrossRef] [PubMed]
8. Tel, A.; Zeppieri, M.; Robiony, M.; Sembronio, S.; Vinayahalingam, S.; Pontoriero, A.; Pergolizzi, S.; Angileri, F.F.; Spadea, L.; Ius, T. Exploring Deep Cervical Compartments in Head and Neck Surgical Oncology through Augmented Reality Vision: A Proof of Concept. *J. Clin. Med.* **2023**, *12*, 6650. [CrossRef] [PubMed]
9. Rose, A.S.; Kim, H.; Fuchs, H.; Frahm, J.M. Development of augmented-reality applications in otolaryngology-head and neck surgery. *Laryngoscope* **2019**, *129* (Suppl. S3), S1–S11. [CrossRef] [PubMed]
10. Salzano, G.; Dell'Aversana Orabona, G.; Abbate, V.; Vaira, L.A.; Committeri, U.; Bonavolontà, P.; Piombino, P.; Maglitto, F.; Russo, C.; Russo, D.; et al. The prognostic role of the pre-treatment neutrophil to lymphocyte ratio (NLR) and tumor depth of invasion (DOI) in early-stage squamous cell carcinomas of the oral tongue. *Oral Maxillofac. Surg.* **2022**, *26*, 21–32. [CrossRef] [PubMed]
11. Taberna, M.; Gil Moncayo, F.; Jané-Salas, E.; Antonio, M.; Arribas, L.; Vilajosana, E.; Peralvez Torres, E.; Mesía, R. The Multidisciplinary Team (MDT) Approach and Quality of Care. *Front. Oncol.* **2020**, *10*, 85. [CrossRef] [PubMed]
12. Garajei, A.; Modarresi, A.; Arabkheradmand, A.; Shirkhoda, M. Functional and esthetic outcomes of virtual surgical planning versus the conventional technique in mandibular reconstruction with a free fibula flap: A retrospective study of 24 cases. *J. Craniomaxillofac. Surg.* **2024**, *52*, 454–463. [CrossRef] [PubMed]

13. Sakkas, A.; Weiß, C.; Zink, W.; Rodriguez, C.A.; Scheurer, M.; Pietzka, S.; Wilde, F.; Thiele, O.C.; Mischkowski, R.A.; Ebeling, M. Airway Management of Orofacial Infections Originating in the Mandible. *J. Pers. Med.* **2023**, *13*, 950. [CrossRef] [PubMed]
14. Gonzalez-Perez, L.-M.; Montes-Carmona, J.-F.; Torres-Carranza, E.; Infante-Cossio, P. Total Joint Replacement for Immediate Reconstruction following Ablative Surgery for Primary Tumors of the Temporo-Mandibular Joint. *J. Pers. Med.* **2023**, *13*, 1021. [CrossRef] [PubMed]
15. Boschetti, C.E.; Vitagliano, R.; Cornacchini, N.; Santagata, M.; Caliendo, V.; Belfiore, M.P.; Colella, G.; Tartaro, G.; Cappabianca, S. Safety and Aesthetics of Autologous Dermis-Fat Graft after Parotidectomy: A Multidisciplinary Retrospective Study. *J. Pers. Med.* **2023**, *13*, 1200. [CrossRef] [PubMed]
16. Ho, J.-P.T.F.; Zhou, N.; van Riet, T.C.T.; Schreurs, R.; Becking, A.G.; de Lange, J. Assessment of Surgical Accuracy in Maxillo-mandibular Advancement Surgery for Obstructive Sleep Apnea: A Preliminary Analysis. *J. Pers. Med.* **2023**, *13*, 1517. [CrossRef] [PubMed]
17. Antúnez-Conde Hidalgo, R.; Silva Canal, J.L.; Navarro Cuéllar, C.; Sánchez Gallego-Albertos, C.; Arias Gallo, J.; Navarro Cuéllar, I.; López Davis, A.; Demaria Martínez, G.; Naranjo Aspas, N.; Zamorano León, J.; et al. Guided Genioplasty: Comparison between Conventional Technique and Customized Guided Surgery. *J. Pers. Med.* **2023**, *13*, 1702. [CrossRef] [PubMed]
18. Serree, P.-E.; Bertin, E.; Coussens, C.; Brumpt, E.; Devoti, J.-F.; Louvrier, A. Assessment of a New Medical Device (PirifixTM) for Positioning and Maintaining the Upper Dental Arch during Le Fort I Osteotomy. *J. Pers. Med.* **2024**, *14*, 324. [CrossRef] [PubMed]
19. Lee, J.-H.; Kim, H.-S.; Park, J.-T. Comparison of Nasal Dimensions According to the Facial and Nasal Indices Using Cone-Beam Computed Tomography. *J. Pers. Med.* **2024**, *14*, 415. [CrossRef] [PubMed]
20. Onică, N.; Budală, D.G.; Baciu, E.-R.; Onică, C.A.; Gelețu, G.L.; Murariu, A.; Balan, M.; Pertea, M.; Stelea, C. Long-Term Clinical Outcomes of 3D-Printed Subperiosteal Titanium Implants: A 6-Year Follow-Up. *J. Pers. Med.* **2024**, *14*, 541. [CrossRef] [PubMed]

Journal of *Personalized Medicine*

Article

Characterization of Tissue Immunity Defense Factors of the Lip in Primary Dentition Children with Bilateral Cleft Lip Palate

Laura Ozola [1,*] and Mara Pilmane [1,2,*]

[1] Institute of Anatomy and Anthropology, Riga Stradins University, Kronvalda Boulevard 9, LV-1010 Riga, Latvia
[2] Children's Clinical University Hospital, Vienības Gatve 45, LV-1004 Riga, Latvia
* Correspondence: laura.ozola@rsu.lv (L.O.); mara.pilmane@rsu.lv (M.P.)

Abstract: Background: Bilateral cleft lip palate is a severe congenital birth defect of the mouth and face. Immunity factors modulate immune response, inflammation, and healing; therefore, they are vital in the assessment of the immunological status of the patient. The aim of this study is to assess the distribution of Gal-10, CD-163, IL-4, IL-6, IL-10, HBD-2, HBD-3, and HBD-4 in tissue of the bilateral cleft lip palate in primary dentition children. Methods: Five patients underwent cheiloplasty surgery, where five tissue samples of lip were obtained. Immunohistochemical staining, semi-quantitative evaluation, and non-parametric statistical analysis were used. Results: A statistically significant increase in HBD-2, HBD-3, and HBD-4 was found in skin and mucosal epithelium, hair follicles, and blood vessels. A notable increase was also noted in IL-4, IL-6, and IL-10 in the mucosal epithelium and CD163 in blood vessels. The connective tissue of patients presented with a statistically significant decrease in Gal-10, IL-10, and HBD-3. Spearman's rank correlation revealed multiple significant positive and negative correlations between the factors. Conclusions: Upregulation of CD163 points to increased angiogenesis but the increase in IL-4 and IL-10 as well as the decrease in Gal-10 points to suppression of excessive inflammatory damage. Decreased connective tissue healing and excessive scarring are suggested by the decrease in HBD-3 and IL-10 and the increase in IL-6.

Keywords: cleft lip and palate; tissue defense factors; primary dentition; HBD; IL; Gal-10; CD-163

1. Introduction

Cleft lip is a type of orofacial cleft defect that affects the upper lip and occasionally the nasal region. It can be unilateral, bilateral, or midline and complete or incomplete [1]. It is two times more common in males than in females and most often affects the left side of the face [1]. Clinically, children with cleft lip have impaired functions of speech, nutrition, and breathing, which significantly decreases the quality of life for the child and for the parents as well as creates a necessity for regular speech therapy, orthodontist, otolaryngology, and nutritionist appointments.

In order to regain symmetry, normal function, and physiological homeostasis of the lip and nasal region, children aged 3 to 4 months undergo surgical correction of the defect [1]. The surgical correction operation is called cheiloplasty, and it is the first of many plastic surgeries that these patients have to undergo in the following years [2]. The first operation focuses on lip repair, and sometimes may include nasoalveolar molding and lip adhesion [2]. Afterward, the surgical correction is followed by definitive cheiloplasty, primary rhinoplasty, palatoplasty, and even orthognathic surgery, all performed when the patient reaches the appropriate age and indications [2].

Afterward, the children are prescribed a strict diet plan in order to limit excessive scarring and possible injury or infection to the site of the operation as well as not to disrupt the remodeling of the tissue [1]; however, due to the constant growth and evolving of the child's orofacial region during this age, asymmetries often occur and a follow-up surgery is necessary to correct the asymmetry [1].

It is also well-known that all orofacial defects have the characteristic feature of chronic inflammation and decreased tissue healing and remodeling potential [3]. However, the fact that cleft lip has a straight connection between the inner and outer environment predisposes the idea that the inflammatory and immune processes in the cleft lip should be much more prominent than in the cleft palate, especially if the cleft lip is bilateral.

Various cells of the immune system produce different proteins for homeostasis maintenance and protection of the tissues, such as anti-inflammatory and regulatory cytokines (interleukin-4, interleukin-10, and interleukin-6) and tissue protective factors (galectin-10 and human beta defensin-2, -3, and -4), complemented by anti-inflammatory M2 macrophages (CD163). The functions of these protective molecules are versatile and, therefore, vital in pathological conditions of the tissues.

Galectin-10 (Gal-10) is a protein that belongs to the prototype class of the galectin family of proteins and contains a specific amino acid sequence that forms the carbohydrate recognition domain [4,5]. Galectin-10 is mainly found in human eosinophils where it is one of the most abundant proteins; however, some traces of it have also been observed in other immune cells like neutrophils, basophils, macrophages, and T cells [5,6]. The functions of galectin-10 are determined by their specific location in eosinophils–immune cells that mainly carry out immune responses targeted to parasites or allergic substances [5,6]. One of the most prominent and important functions of galectin-10 in the immune system is the suppression of T-cell proliferation and receptor activation [7,8]. Therefore, a decrease in Gal-10 can oftentimes increase the count and functions of different subpopulations of T-cells [9]. It has also been noted that increased levels of galectin-10 in pregnancy-related diseases could be connected to the increased development and prolonged maintenance of chronic inflammation via different mutually correlating cytokines and chemokines [5].

CD163 is a distinct hemoglobin scavenger receptor that is expressed by macrophages and monocytes [10]. It is characterized as an important marker for M2 anti-inflammatory macrophages and their activation due to its high specificity to this cell type [11]. Expression of CD163 is induced by IL-6 and IL-10 but decreased by IL-4, TNF-α, IFN-γ, and LPS [11–13]. The main functions of CD163 and M2 macrophages include the secretion of IL-10, NO, and IL-6, improved wound healing and angiogenesis, inhibition of T cells, downregulation of inflammation, and even inhibition of pathogen growth via limited pathogen access to Hb and Fe [12,14].

Interleukin-4 (IL-4) is an inflammatory cytokine that regulates and promotes different inflammatory processes [15]. The main IL-4 secreting cells are T-helper-2 cells (Th2) of the immune system; however, it can also be secreted by basophils, mast cells, T follicular helper cells (Tfh), invariant natural killer T cells (iNKTs), and by eosinophils during allergic reactions or parasitic infections [15,16]. In severe inflammatory processes, IL-4 has multiple functions, mainly focusing on the promotion of tissue repair, reduction in inflammation, and maintenance of tissue homeostasis [17]. Overall, IL-4 has a protective role in tissues to prevent excessive damage caused by the organism's immune response [18].

Interleukin-6 (IL-6) is a pro-inflammatory cytokine that initiates and controls the immune response, inflammatory processes, hematopoiesis, and tissue homeostasis by regulating cytokine production, acute phase protein (ACP) synthesis, cell development, growth, differentiation, activation, and adhesion [19–25]. It is mainly secreted by tissue macrophages and monocytes as a defense mechanism to tissue infections and injuries [23–26]. Excretion of IL-6 has also been observed when cells like fibroblasts, endotheliocytes, epitheliocytes, neutrophils, and lymphocytes come into contact with lipopolysaccharides or inflammatory cytokines, especially IL-1 and TNF-α [24–27]. IL-6 demonstrates both pro- and anti-inflammatory actions and is an important part of the immune response that connects innate and adaptive immune responses and ensures adequate functions of epithelial and mucosal barriers [20,25].

Interleukin-10 (IL-10) is one of the IL-10 family cytokines that has an anti-inflammatory effect and that ensures the suppression of excessive inflammatory responses [28]. It is secreted by the cells of the immune system—T cells (Th1, Th2, Th9, Th17, and Treg), B cells, macrophages, dendritic cells, NK cells, and even CD8+ T cells, eosinophils, and mast cells [28–33]. The most important producer of IL-10 is CD4+ T cells [34]; however, the ability to express IL-10 has also been observed in epithelial cells [28]. IL-10 is also fundamental in the process of healing and wound repair due to the fact that it increases epitheliocyte proliferation, hyaluronan synthesis, re-vascularization, and re-epithelialization [30,35,36].

Human beta-defensins are positively charged antimicrobial peptides that are characterized by their β-sheet structure, expression in the epithelial cells (mainly, keratinocytes), and antimicrobial properties [37–39]. All HBDs except HBD-1 are secreted as a response to inflammation or infection. The main functions of these molecules are the elimination of pathogens, improvement of wound healing, the regulation of inflammation—by controlling cell proliferation, migration, chemotaxis and cytokine production [40–43]. Therefore, they are categorized as the first line of defense of epithelial tissues that ensure immune responses and homeostasis [38,39,44].

Upon release in epithelial tissues, HBD-2 stimulates keratinocyte proliferation and migration, the chemotaxis of macrophages, attraction of T cells and dendritic cells, as well as antimicrobial effects [43,45–47]. Stimulation of cell activity and immune response also ensures wound healing and the epithelial barrier maintenance effects of HBD-2 [43].

The main functions of HBD-3 are the elimination of microbes, stimulation of mast cell degranulation and NK cell activity, increase in chemotaxis and vascular permeability, as well as the stimulation of keratinocyte migration, differentiation, proliferation, and production of IL-6, IL-10, and IFN-γ [41,48–50]. HBD-3 functions not only against Gram-negative bacteria but—unlike other beta-defensins—also against Gram-positive bacteria, therefore ensuring a full spectrum of antibacterial defense [51]. It has also been noted that HBD-3 can prevent the formation of biofilms, especially around various types of implants that have been placed in the body [52]. Overexpression of HBD-3 has been previously linked to increased wound healing and a decreased prevalence of wound infection [41].

The functions of HBD-4 include the stimulation of IL-6, IL-10, IFN-γ, and prostaglandin D_2 production as well as mast cell degranulation and chemotaxis [39,40]. When acting upon bacteria, the antibacterial effect of HBD-4 is carried out by the formation of pores in the cell membrane of these organisms, which is negatively charged [37].

In summary, the main functions and properties of the described cytokines and factors are as follows: IL-6 is a regulatory cytokine of other cytokines; IL-4 is a dual anti- and pro-inflammatory cytokine; IL-10 is the strongest anti-inflammatory cytokine; M2 are anti-inflammatory macrophages; HBDs are protective molecules of the tissues; and the role of Gal-10 is still unclear, although its functions are mainly expressed in eosinophilic inflammation. Little is known about the correlations and links between these molecules in different pathological states of the tissues.

Due to the fact that local tissue defense factors are crucial mediators of inflammation, the immune response, tissue healing, and remodeling, they have been previously researched in various other studies trying to connect them with the pathological characteristics of certain conditions, including pathologies of the oral and maxillofacial region like nasal polyps, periodontitis, and various types of clefts.

The aim of this study is to assess the distribution of tissue defense factors and detect the local tissue defense status in the bilateral cleft lip and palate in children of primary dentition since prominent features of the BCLP are chronic inflammation and insufficient healing. The results of this study will continue to be a part of a continuous research cycle in order to find possible links and causalities between defense factors and characteristics of clefted tissue.

2. Materials and Methods

2.1. Material Characteristics of Subjects

This research was conducted in accordance with the 1975 Helsinki Declaration (as revised in 2008). This study was independently reviewed and approved by the Ethical Committee of the Riga Stradiņš University (22 May 2003; 17 January 2013; Nr. 5/28 June

2018). All parents of the patients were fully informed about the nature of this study, and they provided written informed consent for participation in the study and its publication.

2.2. Selection Criteria of Patient Tissue Samples

Samples were selected according to the following inclusion criteria:

- Diagnosis of Cheilognathouranoschisis bilateralis;
- Age of primary dentition;
- No other congenital diseases;
- Absence of additional pathologies that are contraindications to cheiloplasty;
- No signs of active inflammation
- Indications for bilateral cheiloplasty.
- The following exclusion criteria were also applied:
- Age during primary dentition [53];
- Presence of other congenital diseases;
- Contraindicative pathologies for plastic surgery;
- Signs of active inflammation.

2.3. Characteristics of Selected Patients

Four of the selected patients were male and one was female. One patient's mother had refused to take mandatory pregnancy medication during pregnancy and another patient's mother had a history of cleft (Table 1). All patients underwent bilateral cheiloplasty surgery.

Table 1. Description of the patients.

Patient Number	Age (Months)	Sex	Remarks
238	4	M	
264	4	F	
396	4	F	Mother did not use medication during pregnancy
395	6	F	Mother with a cleft
369	17	F	

Abbreviations: M—male; F—female.

In total, 5 patient samples of lip tissue were obtained during cheiloplasty surgery in the Cleft Lip and Palate Centre of the Institute of Stomatology of Riga Stradins University. The samples were acquired from children aged 4 to 17 months old that were diagnosed with bilateral cleft lip (Cheilognathouranoschisis bilateralis).

2.4. Selection Criteria of Control Tissue Samples

The inclusion criteria for the control group were as follows:

- Absence of craniofacial clefts in patient examination, anamnesis, and/or family history;
- Absence of additional pathologies, congenital abnormalities, or damage of oral cavity tissue.

In total, 5 control tissue samples were obtained from the Institute of Anatomy and Anthropology of Riga Stradins University during post-mortem necropsies.

One of the selected control samples was male and four were female. The age of the control group samples varied from newborn to 24 weeks old. Two of the controls were affected by asphyxia of the umbilical cord, two by sudden death syndrome, and one was aborted due to the health status of the mother (Table 2).

The approval Nr. 2-PEK-4/595/2022 for the use of control group tissue was issued on 14 December 2022.

Table 2. Description of the control group.

Control Number	Age	Sex	Cause of Death
1a	Newborn	M	Birth asphyxia
2a	Newborn	F	Birth asphyxia
4a	24 weeks old	F	Abortion due to the maternal indication
5a	Newborn	F	Sudden infant death syndrome
6a	Newborn	F	Sudden infant death syndrome

Abbreviations: M—male; F—female.

2.5. Routine Staining

Firstly, the obtained tissue material was fixated for 24 h using 2% formaldehyde, 0.2% picric acid, and 0.1 M phosphate buffer (pH 7.2). Secondly, the material was processed for 12 h using Tyrode's buffer with 10% saccharose. Thirdly, embedding of the tissues in paraffin and cutting with microtome into 5–7 µm sections was performed. Lastly, the prepared lip tissue samples were stained with hematoxylin and eosin [54].

2.6. Immunohistochemical (IHC) Analysis

Immunohistochemical detection of the local tissue defense factor quantity in the selected lip tissue samples was performed using the standard streptavidin and biotin method [54,55].

Firstly, antibodies were diluted in antibody diluent (code-938B-05, Cell Marque™, Rocklin, CA, USA).

Secondly, tissue samples were prepared for the antibodies: previously cut tissue sections were deparaffinized, washed in alcohol and water, rinsed with TRIS buffer solution (code-2017X12508, Diapath S.p.A., Martinengo, Italy) twice for 5 min, placed in a microwave with boiling EDTA buffer (code-2017X02239, Diapath S.p.A., Martinengo, Italy) for 20 min, and cooled. Then, the samples were once again washed with TRIS buffer two times for 5 min, blocked with 3% peroxide for 10 min, and washed with TRIS buffer.

Thirdly, the antibody reaction was performed: samples were incubated with primary antibodies for 1 h, washed 3 times with TRIS buffer, exposed to HiDef Detection™ reaction amplificator (code 954D-31, Cell Marque™, Rocklin, CA, USA) for 10 min at room temperature, washed with TRIS buffer, incubated with a HiDef DetectionTM HRP Polymer Detector (code-954D-32, Cell Marque™, Rocklin, CA, USA) for 10 min at room temperature, followed by the last wash with TRIS buffer 3 times for 5 min each.

Lastly, the samples were prepared for sealing: tissue was coated with a DAB+ chromogenic liquid DAB Substrate Kit (code 957D-60, Cell Marque™, Rocklin, CA, USA) for 10 min, rinsed with running water, counterstained with hematoxylin (code-05-M06002, Mayer's Hematoxylin, Bio Optica Milano S.p.A., Milano, Italy), dehydrated with ethanol of increasing concentrations (70°–90°), clarified with carboxylic acid and xylol, sealed with a coverslip, and marked according to the patient number and antibody used.

The information about the antibodies used is summarized in Table 3.

Table 3. Information about the antibodies used in IHC.

Tissue Factor	Product Code	Working Dilution	Company	Location
Gal-10	ab157475	1:200	Abcam	Cambridge, UK
CD 163	ab87099	1:200	Abcam	Cambridge, UK
IL-4	orb10908	1:100	Biorbyt	Cambridge, UK
IL-6	sc-28343	1:100	Santa Cruz Biotechnology Inc.	Santa Cruz, CA, USA
IL-10	orb100193	1:600	Biorbyt LLC	St Louis, MO, USA
HBD-2	sc-20798	1:100	Santa Cruz Biotechnology Inc.	Dallas, TX, USA
HBD-3	orb183268	1:100	Biorbyt LLC	St Louis, MO, USA
HBD-4	ab70215	1:100	Abcam	Cambridge, UK

2.7. Assessment of Local Tissue Defense Factor Quantity

Light microscopy and the semi-quantitative counting method were used to assess the relative quantity of Gal-10-, CD-163-, IL-4-, IL-6-, IL-10-, HBD-2-, HBD-3-, and HBD-4-positive structures in skin and the mucosal epithelium, connective tissue and blood vessels, salivary and adipose gland ducts, and hair follicles. Evaluation of positively stained structures visible in the visual field was performed according to identifiers summarized in Table 4. Acquisition, processing, and analyses of the tissue sample pictures were performed using a Leica DC 300F digital camera (Leica Microsystems Digital Imaging, Cambridge, UK) and the Image Pro Plus program (Media Cybernetics, Inc., Rockville, MD, USA).

Table 4. Explanation of semi-quantitative evaluation identifiers [56,57].

Identifier Used	Explanation
0	No positive structures (0%)
0/+	Rare occurrence of positive structures (12.5%)
+	Few positive structures (25%)
+/++	Few to moderate number of positive structures (37.5%)
++	Moderate number of positive structures (50%)
++/+++	Moderate to numerous positive structures (62.5%)
+++	Numerous positive structures (75%)
+++/++++	Numerous to abundant positive structures (87.5%)
++++	Abundance of positive structures (100%)

2.8. Statistical Analysis

IBM SPSS (Statistical Package for the Social Sciences) software version 26.0 (IBM Company, Chicago, IL, USA) was used for statistical processing of the data. Statistical significance was selected at a p-value < 0.05 and was used for every statistical assessment of the tests and results [58]. Semi-quantitative evaluation of the local tissue defense factor quantity produced ordinal data (non-numeric and arranged in a specific and unchangeable order); therefore, descriptive statistics, analytical statistics, and non-parametric tests were used to calculate the results and their statistical significance.

2.8.1. Mann–Whitney U Test

This test was used to detect if the distribution of immunity factor quantity in the patient and control group samples was equal or not, and if the difference was statistically significant [58].

2.8.2. Spearman's Rank Correlation

This test was used to detect whether there was a statistically significant rate of connection between changes in one factor that was connected to the changes in another factor [58]. The strength of the correlation between factors was interpreted using the following definition of Spearman's rho (r_s) values:

- A very weak correlation: r_s = 0.00–0.19;
- A weak correlation: r_s = 0.20–0.39;
- A moderate correlation: r_s = 0.40–0.59;
- A strong correlation: r_s = 0.60–0.79;
- A very strong correlation: r_s = 0.80–1.00 [59].

2.9. Flowchart

A visual summary of the workflow and information presented in the Materials and Methods Section is outlined in Figure 1.

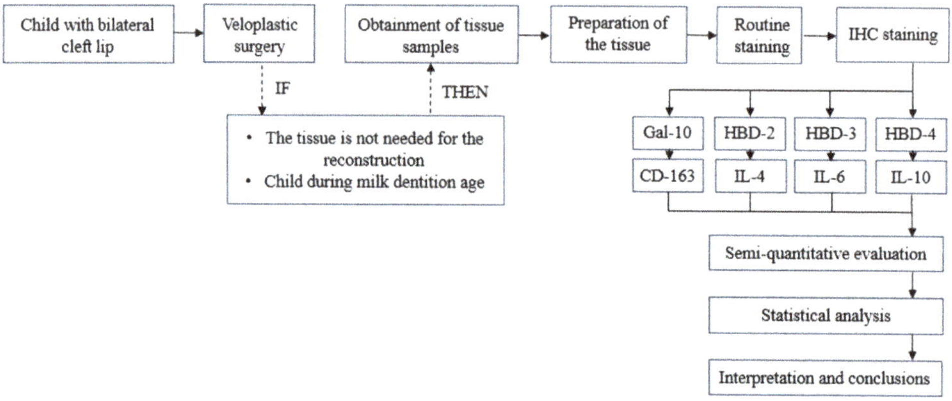

Figure 1. Workflow of patient tissue sample selection, processing, and research.

3. Results

3.1. Characteristics of Routine Staining

The control sample showed features of normal lip tissue—non-keratinized stratified squamous mucosal epithelium, keratinized stratified squamous skin epithelium with sweat gland ducts and hair follicles, and underlying mucosal connective tissue with adipose glands. The patient tissue samples presented with prominent epithelial vacuolization and subepithelial infiltration of inflammatory cells (Figure 2a,b).

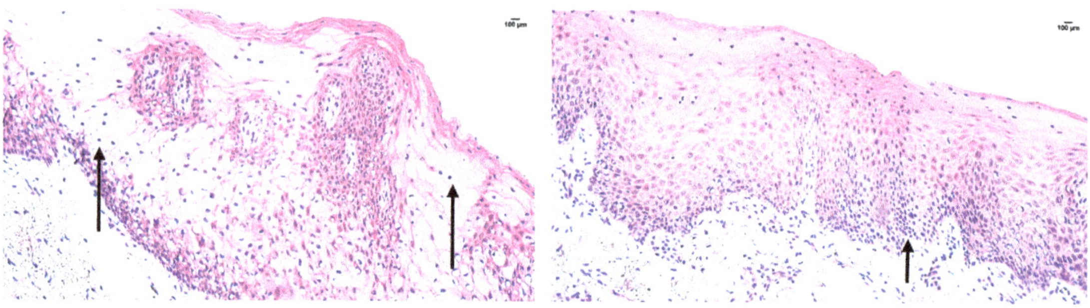

(**a**) (**b**)

Figure 2. Hematoxylin and eosin routine staining of the patient tissue samples (**a**,**b**): note vacuolization (**a**) and inflammatory cell infiltration (**b**) in skin type epithelium of the lip (arrows). Magnification 200×.

3.2. Appearance and Distribution of Gal-10

In the control group, the median quantity of Gal-10-positive structures was moderate (++) in the mucosal epithelium, blood vessels, sweat gland ducts, hair follicles, and connective tissue, moderate to numerous (++/+++) in the skin epithelium, and numerous (+++) in adipose glands (Figure 3a, Table 5).

In the patient group, the median quantity of Gal-10-positive structures was few to moderate (+/++) in blood vessels, moderate (++) in sweat gland ducts and hair follicles, moderate to numerous (++/+++) in skin epithelium and adipose glands, and none in connective tissue (Figure 3b, Table 5).

Comparison of both groups using the Mann–Whitney U test illustrates a statistically significant difference (U = 0, p = 0.005) in the connective tissue (Table 6). In addition, there were no statistically significant differences in the skin epithelium (U = 10, p = 0.589), mucosal epithelium (U = 6.5, p = 0.368), blood vessels (U = 5.0, p = 0.199), sweat gland ducts (U = 2.0, p = 0.414), adipose glands (U = 3.5, p = 0.803), and hair follicles (U = 2.5, p = 0.195) (Table 6).

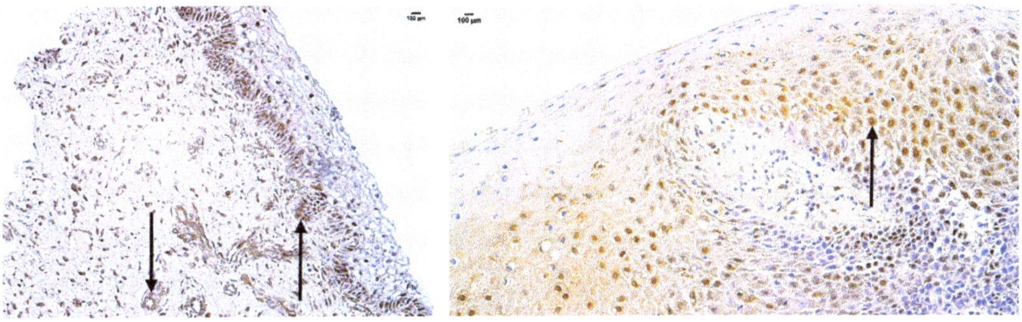

(**a**) (**b**)

Figure 3. Immunohistochemistry of the Gal-10-positive structures in the control and patient tissue samples: (**a**) control sample with moderate to numerous Gal-10-positive structures in skin epithelium, and moderate in mucosal epithelium, sweat gland ducts, and connective tissue (arrows), 200×; (**b**) patient sample with few to moderate Gal-10-positive structures in blood vessels, moderate to numerous in skin epithelium, and numerous in mucosal epithelium (arrows), 200×.

Table 5. Semi-quantitative evaluation of Gal-10 and CD-163 in control and patient groups.

Sample Number	Gal-10							CD-163						
	SE	ME	BV	SG	AG	F	CT	SE	ME	BV	SG	AG	F	CT
396	+/++	++/+++	+	++	+++	+	0	0	0	+	+++	++	0/+	++
369	++/+++	-	++	++	++	++	0/+	+	0	+/++	+	+/++	0/+	++
395	++/+++	+++	+/++	-	-	-	0	0/+	0/+	+	+	-	+	+
264	++	+++	0/+	-	-	-	0	+	0/+	++/+++	+	-	-	++/+++
238	++/+++	+++	+++	+++	-	+++	0	++	+/++	++	++	-	++	++
Patient Median	++/+++	+++	+/++	++	++/+++	++	0	+	0/+	+/++	+	++	+	++
1a	+	+	++	-	++/+++	+++	++	0	0	0/+	-	-	0	+
2a	++++	+	++	-	++	+++	++	0	0/+	+	0/+	-	-	++
4a	+++/++++	+++/++++	+++	-	-	++++	++/+++	+	+/++	+	+	-	-	++
5a	++/+++	++		++	+++	-	++	0	-	+	+	-	-	++
6a	++	+++	++	++	+++	++	++	0	0	0	-	0	0	0
Control Median	++/+++	++	++	++	+++	++	++	0	0/+	+	+	0	0	++

Abbreviations: SE—skin epithelium; ME—mucosal epithelium; BV—blood vessels; SG—salivary glands; AG—adipose glands; F—hair follicles; CT—connective tissue; Gal-10—galectin-10.

Table 6. Median values for Gal-10 and CD-163 in patient and control groups.

	Gal-10							CD-163						
	SE	ME	BV	SG	AG	F	CT	SE	ME	BV	SG	AG	F	CT
P	++/+++	+++	+/++	++	++/+++	++	0	+	0/+	+/++	+	++	+	++
C	++/+++	++	++	++	+++	++	++	0	0/+	+	+	0	0	++
U-test value	10.0	6.5	5.0	2.0	3.5	2.5	0.0	5.0	9.5	3.0	3.0	0.0	0.0	8.0
p-value	0.589	0.368	0.199	0.414	0.803	0.195	0.005	0.090	0.896	0.034	0.124	0.221	0.057	0.288

Abbreviations: SE—skin epithelium; ME—mucosal epithelium; BV—blood vessels; SG—salivary glands; AG—adipose glands; F—hair follicles; CT—connective tissue; Gal-10—galectin-10.

3.3. Appearance and Distribution of CD-163

In the control group, the median quantity of CD-163-positive structures was none (0) in lip skin epithelium or around adipose glands and hair follicles, rare (0/+) in the mucosal epithelium, few (+) in the blood vessels and sweat gland ducts, and moderate (++) in connective tissue (Figure 4a, Table 5).

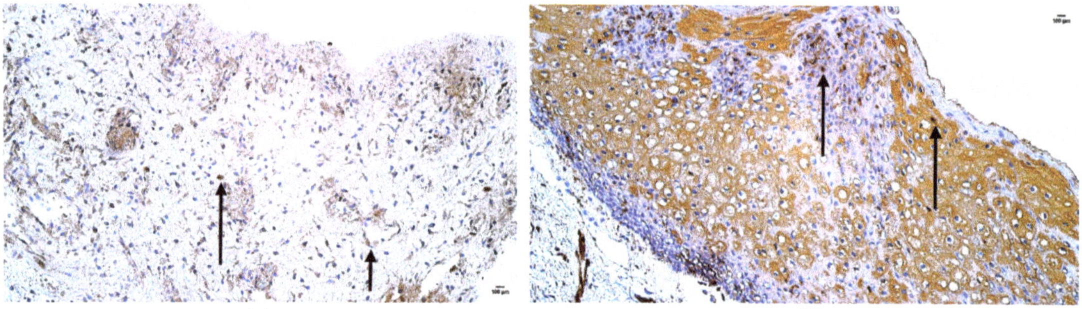

(**a**) (**b**)

Figure 4. Immunohistochemistry of the CD-163-positive structures in the control and patient tissue samples: (**a**) control sample with rare occurrence of CD-163-positive structures in mucosal epithelium and sweat gland ducts, few in the blood vessels, and moderate in connective tissue (arrows), 200×; (**b**) patient sample with few to moderate CD-163-positive structures in mucosal epithelium and moderate in the skin epithelium (arrows), 200×.

In the patient group, the median quantity of CD-163-positive structures was rare (0/+) in the mucosal epithelium, few (+) in skin epithelium, sweat gland ducts, and hair follicles, few to moderate (+/++) in blood vessels, and moderate (++) in adipose glands and connective tissue (Figure 4b, Table 5).

Comparison of both groups using the Mann–Whitney U test illustrates a statistically significant difference (U = 3.0, p = 0.034) in the blood vessels. (Table 6). In addition, no statistically significant differences in skin epithelium (U = 5.0, p = 0.090), mucosal epithelium (U = 9.5, p = 0.896), sweat gland ducts (U = 3.0, p = 0.124), adipose glands (U =0, p = 0.221), and connective tissue (U = 8.0, p = 0.288) were found (Table 6).

3.4. Appearance and Distribution of IL-4

In the control group, the median quantity of IL-4-positive structures was none (0) in the skin epithelium, sweaty glands, and connective tissue, rare (0/+) in adipose glands, hair follicles, and mucosal epithelium, and few to moderate (+/++) in blood vessels (Figure 5a, Table 7).

Table 7. Semi-quantitative evaluation of IL-4 and IL-6 in control and patient groups.

Sample Number	IL-4							IL-6						
	SE	ME	BV	SG	AG	F	CT	SE	ME	BV	SG	AG	F	CT
396	+	+++	0	++	0/+	+	0	+	+++	+	+++	+++	+/++	++
369	0	-	0	+	0/+	0/+	0	++	-	++	++	++	++	++
395	++	++/+++	-	-	-	-	0	+++	+++/++++	0/+	-	-	-	++
264	+	++/+++	0	-	-	-	+	++	++/+++	+/++	++	-	-	++/+++
238	++	+++	0/+	++/+++	-	++/+++	+	++/+++	+++/++++	++/+++	++/+++	-	+++	++/+++
Patient Median	+	+++	0	++	0/+	+	0	++	+++/++++	+/++	++/+++	++/+++	++	++
1a	0	0/+	-	-	0/+	+/++	0	+	+	0/+	-	-	++	+
2a	0	0/+	-	-	0	0/+	0	+	+	++	-	-	++/+++	+/++
4a	-	0/+	-	-	0/+	0/+	-	++	-	++/+++	-	+++	+++	++
5a	-	0/+	+/++	-	-	+	-	+	-	++	++	-	-	++
6a	0	0	-	0	0	0	0	++	++	++	-	++	++	++
Control Median	0	0/+	+/++	0	0/+	0/+	0	+	+	++	++	++/+++	++/+++	++

Abbreviations: SE—skin epithelium; ME—mucosal epithelium; BV—blood vessels; SG—salivary glands; AG—adipose glands; F—hair follicles; CT—connective tissue; IL-4—interleukin-4; IL-6—interleukin-6.

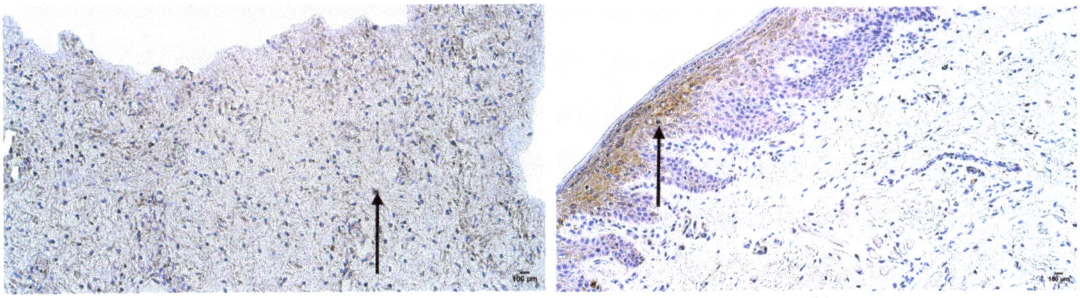

(a) (b)

Figure 5. Immunohistochemistry of the IL-4-positive structures in the control and patient tissue samples: (**a**) control sample with no IL-4-positive structures in skin and mucosal epithelium and adipose glands, with rare occurrence in blood vessels, hair follicles, and connective tissue (arrows), 200×; (**b**) patient sample with few IL-4-positive structures in skin epithelium and connective tissue (arrows), 200×.

In the patient group, the median quantity of IL-4-positive structures was none (0) in the blood vessels and connective tissue, rare (0/+) in adipose glands, few (+) in skin epithelium and hair follicles, moderate (++) in sweat gland ducts, and numerous (+++) in the mucosal epithelium (Figure 5b, Table 7).

Comparison of both groups using the Mann–Whitney U test illustrates a statistically significant difference (U = 0, p = 0.025) in the mucosal epithelium (Table 8). In addition, no statistically significant differences in skin epithelium (U = 4.0, p = 0.054), blood vessels (U = 4.5, p = 0.120), sweat gland ducts (U = 1.0, p = 0.655), adipose glands (U = 0, p = 0.157), hair follicles (U = 1.0, p = 0.064), and connective tissue (U = 8.5, p = 0.381) were found (Table 8).

Table 8. Median values for IL-4 and IL-6 in patient and control groups.

	IL-4							IL-6						
	SE	**ME**	**BV**	**SG**	**AG**	**F**	**CT**	**SE**	**ME**	**BV**	**SG**	**AG**	**F**	**CT**
P	+	+++	0	++	0/+	+	0	++	+++/++++	+/++	++/+++	++/+++	++	++
C	0	0/+	+/++	0	0/+	0/+	0	+	+	++	++	++/+++	++/+++	++
U-test value	4.0	0.0	4.5	1.0	0.0	1.0	8.5	5.5	0.0	9.5	1.0	2.0	4.5	4.5
p-value	0.054	0.025	0.120	0.655	0.157	0.064	0.381	0.119	0.031	0.515	0.429	1.000	0.578	0.059

Abbreviations: SE—skin epithelium; ME—mucosal epithelium; BV—blood vessels; SG—salivary glands; AG—adipose glands; F—hair follicles; CT—connective tissue; IL-4—interleukin-4; IL-6—interleukin-6.

3.5. *Appearance and Distribution of IL-6*

In the control group, the median quantity of IL-6-positive structures was few (+) in the skin epithelium and mucosal epithelium, moderate (++) in blood vessels, sweat gland ducts, and connective tissue, and moderate to numerous (++/+++) in adipose glands and hair follicles (Figure 6a, Table 7).

In the patient group, the median quantity of Gal-10-positive structures was few to moderate (+/++) in the blood vessels, moderate (++) in skin epithelium, hair follicles, and connective tissue, moderate to numerous (++/+++) in sweat gland ducts and adipose glands, and numerous to abundant (+++/++++) in the mucosal epithelium (Figure 6b, Table 7).

Comparison of both groups using the Mann–Whitney U test illustrates a statistically significant difference (U = 0, p = 0.031) in the mucosal epithelium (Table 8). In addition, no statistically significant differences in skin epithelium (U = 5.5, p = 0.119), blood vessels (U = 9.5, p = 0.515), sweat gland ducts (U = 1.0, p = 0.429), adipose glands (U = 2.0, p = 1.000), hair follicles (U = 4.5, $p = 0.578$), and connective tissue (U = 4.5, $p = 0.059$) were found (Table 8).

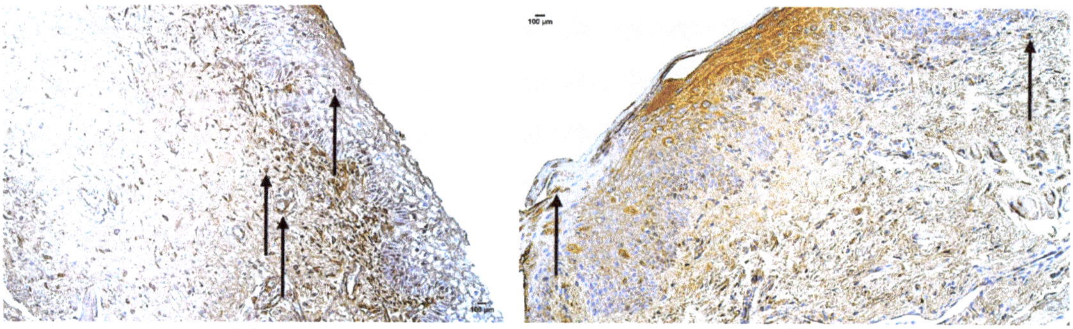

(a) (b)

Figure 6. Immunohistochemistry of the IL-6-positive structures in the control and patient tissue samples: (**a**) control sample with few IL-6-positive structures in the skin epithelium and moderate in the blood vessels, sweat gland ducts, and connective tissue (arrows), 200×; (**b**) patient sample with few to moderate IL-6-positive structures in blood vessels, with moderate in skin epithelium and sweat gland ducts, and moderate to numerous in mucosal epithelium and connective tissue (arrows), 200×.

3.6. Appearance and Distribution of HBD-2

In the control group, the median quantity of HBD-2-positive structures was none (0) in the skin epithelium, blood vessels, adipose glands, and connective tissue, and rare (0/+) in the mucosal epithelium, sweat gland ducts, and hair follicles (Figure 7a, Table 9).

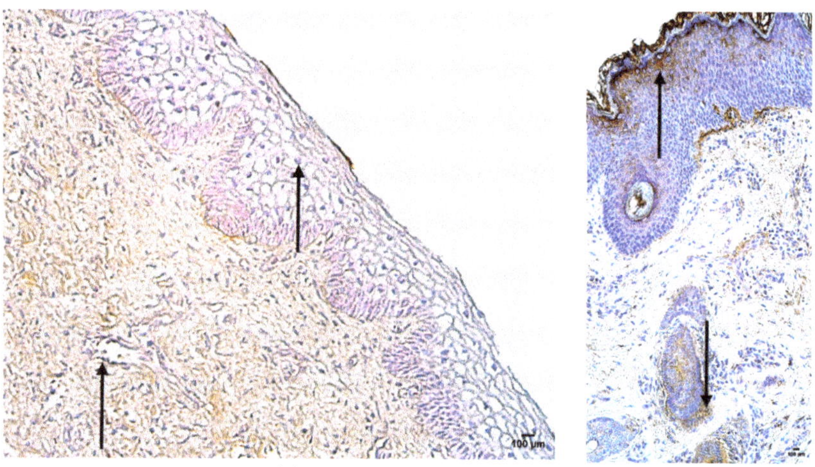

(a) (b)

Figure 7. Immunohistochemistry of the HBD-2-positive structures in the control and patient tissue samples: (**a**) control sample with the absence of HBD-2-positive structures in skin epithelium, blood vessels, and connective tissue (arrows), 200×; (**b**) patient sample with rare occurrence of HBD-2-positive structures in connective tissue, moderate to numerous in skin epithelium and adipose glands, and numerous to abundant in mucosal epithelium (arrows), 200×.

Table 9. Semi-quantitative evaluation of HBD-2 and HBD-3 in control and patient groups.

Sample Number	HBD-2							HBD-3						
	SE	ME	BV	SG	AG	F	CT	SE	ME	BV	SG	AG	F	CT
396	+/++	+++	+	++/+++	++	+	0/+	0/+	+++	++	++	+++	++/+++	0/+
369	+/++	-	+/++	+	0/+	+	0	++	-	++	-	++	++	++
395	++/+++	+++/++++	0	-	++/+++	-	0/+	+++	+++/++++	0	-	-	-	0
264	++/+++	++	+/++	+	++	-	0/+	++	++	+	0/+	-	-	0/+
238	+/++	+	++	++	-	++	+/++	+/++	++	+/++	+++/++++	+++	+++	0/+
Patient Median	+/++	++/+++	+/++	+/++	++	+	0/+	++	++/+++	+/++	++	+++	++/+++	0/+
1a	0	0/+	0	-	-	0/+	0	+	+	+	-	+/++	++/+++	++
2a	0/+	0/+	0/+	-	0	0/+	0/+	+	+	+/++	-	++	++/+++	+++
4a	0/+	-	0	-	0	0	0	+/++	+/++	++	-	+++	+++	++/+++
5a	0	-	0	0/+	-	-	0	0/+	-	+	+/++	-	-	++
6a	0	0	0	0/+	-	0	0	+/++	+/++	+/++	+	++	++	++
Control Median	0	0/+	0	0/+	0	0/+	0	+	+/++	+/++	+/++	++	++/+++	++

Abbreviations: SE—skin epithelium; ME—mucosal epithelium; BV—blood vessels; SG—salivary glands; AG—adipose glands; F—hair follicles; CT—connective tissue; HBD-2—human beta-defensin 2; HBD-3—human beta-defensin 3.

In the patient group, the median quantity of HBD-2-positive structures was few (+) in the hair follicles, few to moderate (+/++) in skin epithelium, blood vessels, and sweat gland ducts, moderate (++) in adipose glands, and moderate to numerous (++/+++) in the mucosal epithelium (Figure 7b, Table 9).

Comparison of both groups using the Mann–Whitney U test illustrates statistically significant differences in skin epithelium (U = 0, p = 0.007), mucosal epithelium (U = 0, p = 0.032), blood vessels (U = 3.0, p = 0.034), and hair follicles (U = 0, p = 0.029) (Table 10). In addition, no statistically significant differences in the sweat gland ducts (U = 0, p = 0.057), adipose glands (U = 0, p = 0.057), and connective tissue (U = 0, p = 0.007) were found (Table 10).

Table 10. Median values for HBD-2 and HBD-3 in patient and control groups.

	HBD-2							HBD-3						
	SE	ME	BV	SG	AG	F	CT	SE	ME	BV	SG	AG	F	CT
P	+/++	++/+++	+/++	+/++	++	+	0/+	++	++/+++	+/++	++	+++	++/+++	0/+
C	0	0/+	0	0/+	0	0/+	0	+	+/++	+/++	+/++	++	++/+++	++
U-test value	0.0	0.0	3.0	0.0	0.0	0.0	0.0	5.5	0.0	12.0	2.0	3.0	6.0	1.5
p-value	0.007	0.032	0.034	0.057	0.057	0.029	0.007	0.135	0.019	0.914	0.564	0.252	1.000	0.016

Abbreviations: SE—skin epithelium; ME—mucosal epithelium; BV—blood vessels; SG—salivary glands; AG—adipose glands; F—hair follicles; CT—connective tissue; HBD-2—human beta-defensin 2; HBD-3—human beta-defensin 3.

3.7. Appearance and Distribution of HBD-3

In the control group, the median quantity of HBD-3-positive structures was few (+) in the skin epithelium, few to moderate (+/++) in the mucosal epithelium, blood vessels, and sweat gland ducts, moderate (++) in the adipose glands and connective tissue, and moderate to numerous (++/+++) in hair follicles (Figure 8a, Table 9).

In the patient group, the median quantity of HBD-3-positive structures was rare (0/+) in the connective tissue, few to moderate (+/++) in blood vessels, moderate (++) in skin epithelium and sweat glands, moderate to numerous (++/+++) in the mucosal epithelium and hair follicles, and numerous (+++) in adipose glands (Figure 8b, Table 9).

Comparison of both groups using the Mann–Whitney U test illustrates statistically significant differences in mucosal epithelium (U = 0, p = 0.019) and connective tissue (U = 1.5, p = 0.016) (Table 10). In addition, no statistically significant differences in the skin epithelium (U = 5.5, p = 0.135), blood vessels (U = 12.0, p = 0.914), sweat gland ducts (U = 2.0, p = 0.564), adipose glands (U = 3.0, p = 0.252), and hair follicles (U = 6.0, p = 1.000) were found (Table 10).

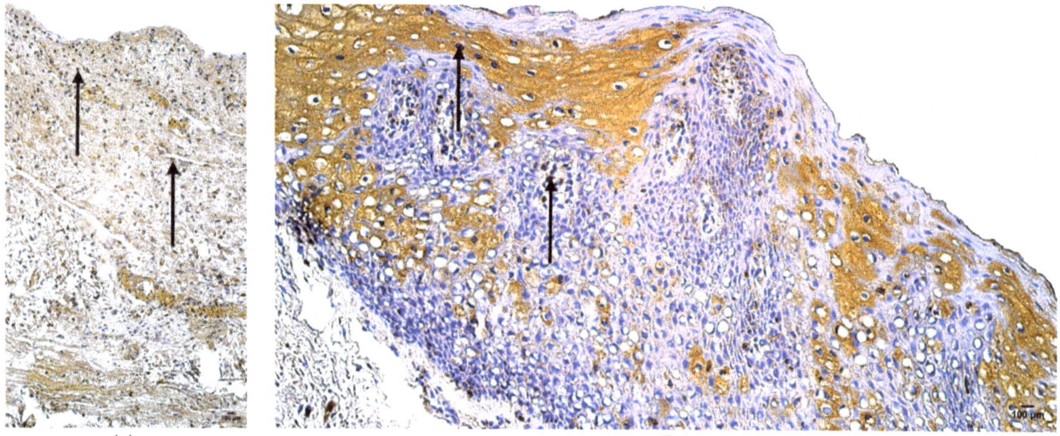

(**a**) (**b**)

Figure 8. Immunohistochemistry of the HBD-3-positive structures in the control and patient tissue samples: (**a**) control sample with few HBD-3-positive structures in skin and mucosal epithelium, few to moderate in blood vessels, numerous in adipose glands, moderate to numerous in hair follicles, numerous in connective tissue (arrows), 200×; (**b**) patient sample with rare HBD-3-positive structures in connective tissue, few to moderate in blood vessels and skin epithelium, moderate in mucosal epithelium, numerous in adipose glands and hair follicles, numerous to abundant in sweat gland ducts (arrows), 200×.

3.8. Appearance and Distribution of HBD-4

In the control group, the median quantity of HBD-4-positive structures was rare (0/+) in the blood vessels and connective tissue, few to moderate (+/++) in sweat gland ducts, moderate (++) in skin epithelium and adipose glands, moderate to numerous (++/+++) in hair follicles, and numerous (+++) in the mucosal epithelium (Figure 9a, Table 11).

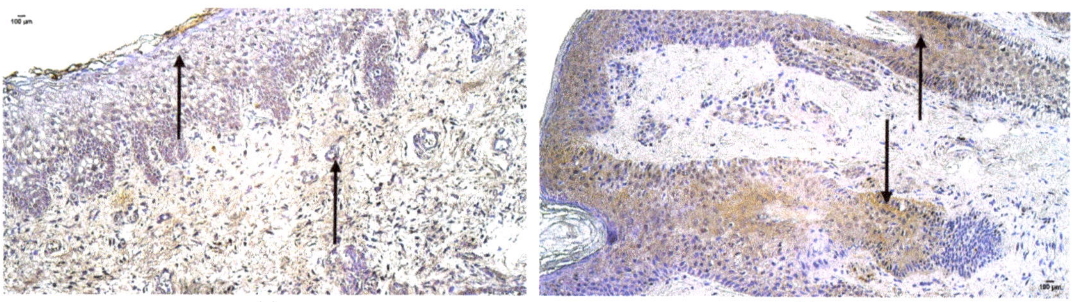

(**a**) (**b**)

Figure 9. Immunohistochemistry of the HBD-4-positive structures in the control and patient tissue samples: (**a**) control sample with no HBD-4-positive structures in skin and mucosal epithelium, adipose glands, hair follicles, and connective tissue, rare in blood vessels (arrows), 200×; (**b**) patient sample with rare HBD-4-positive structures in blood vessels and connective tissue, moderate in skin epithelium, moderate to numerous in adipose glands and hair follicles, numerous in mucosal epithelium and sweat gland ducts (arrows), 200×.

Table 11. Semi-quantitative evaluation of HBD-4 and IL-10 in control and patient groups.

Sample Number	HBD-4							IL-10						
	SE	ME	BV	SG	AG	F	CT	SE	ME	BV	SG	AG	F	CT
396	++	+++	0/+	+++	++/+++	++/+++	0/+	+	+++	++	++/+++	++/+++	0/+	+
369	+	-	++	+/++	+	++	0/+	+	-	+	++	0/+	+/++	0/+
395	++/+++	+++	0	-	-	-	0	++/+++	+++	++	-	-	-	+
264	++	++	0/+	0/+	-	-	0/+	++	+/++	0/+	-	-	+	+
238	++	+++	0/+	-	-	++/+++	+	+	+++	++	+++	-	++	+/++
Patient Median	++	+++	0/+	+/++	++	++/+++	0/+	+	+++	++	++/+++	+/++	+/++	+
1a	0	0	0/+	-	0	0/+	0	++	++	+/++	-	-	+++	+++
2a	0	0	0/+	0	0/+	0/+	0	++	+	++	-	++	++	+++
4a	0	0	0/+	-	0	0	0	+	0/+	+	-	0	0/+	++/+++
5a	0	-	0	0	-	-	0	0/+	-	+/++	0/+	-	-	++/+++
6a	+	0/+	0/+	-	0/+	+	0/+	++	+	+	-	0/+	++	++
Control Median	0	0	0/+	0	0/+	0/+	0	++	+	+/++	0/+	0/+	++	++/+++

Abbreviations: SE—skin epithelium; ME—mucosal epithelium; BV—blood vessels; SG—salivary glands; AG—adipose glands; F—hair follicles; CT—connective tissue; HBD-4—human beta-defensin 4; IL-10—interleukin-10.

In the patient group, the median quantity of HBD-4-positive structures was none (0) in the skin epithelium, mucosal epithelium, sweat gland ducts, and connective tissue, and rare (0/+) in blood vessels, adipose glands, and hair follicles (Figure 9b, Table 11).

Comparison of both groups using the Mann–Whitney U test illustrates statistically significant differences in the skin epithelium (U = 0.5, p = 0.009), mucosal epithelium (U = 0, p = 0.015), and hair follicles (U = 0, p = 0.031) (Table 12). In addition, no statistically significant differences in blood vessels (U = 10.5, p = 0.606), sweat gland ducts (U = 0, p = 0.076), adipose glands (U = 0, p = 0.057), and connective tissue (U = 4.5, p = 0.065) were found (Table 12).

Table 12. Median values for HBD-4 and IL-10 in patient and control groups.

	HBD-4							IL-10						
	SE	ME	BV	SG	AG	F	CT	SE	ME	BV	SG	AG	F	CT
P	++	+++	0/+	+/++	++	++/+++	0/+	+	+++	++	++/+++	+/++	+/++	+
C	0	0	0/+	0	0/+	0/+	0	++	+	+/++	0/+	0/+	++	++/+++
U-test value	0.5	0.0	10.5	0.0	0.0	0.0	4.5	12.0	1.0	10.5	0.0	1.5	4.5	0.0
p-value	0.009	0.015	0.606	0.076	0.057	0.031	0.065	0.911	0.037	0.661	0.180	0.374	0.297	0.008

Abbreviations: SE—skin epithelium; ME—mucosal epithelium; BV—blood vessels; SG—salivary glands; AG—adipose glands; F—hair follicles; CT—connective tissue; HBD-4—human beta-defensin 4; IL-10—interleukin-10.

3.9. *Appearance and Distribution of IL-10*

In the control group, the median quantity of CD-163-positive structures was rare (0/+) in the sweat gland ducts and adipose glands, few (0) in the mucosal epithelium, few to moderate (+/++) in blood vessels, moderate (++) in skin epithelium and hair follicles, and moderate to numerous (++/+++) in connective tissue (Figure 10a, Table 11).

In the patient group, the median quantity of IL-10-positive structures was few (+) in the skin epithelium and connective tissue, few to moderate (+/++) in adipose glands and hair follicles, moderate (++) in blood vessels, moderate to numerous (++/+++) in sweat gland ducts, and numerous (+++) in the mucosal epithelium (Figure 10b, Table 11).

Comparison of both groups with the Mann–Whitney U test illustrates statistically significant differences in the mucosal epithelium (U = 1.0, p = 0.037) and connective tissue (U = 0, p = 0.008) (Table 12). In addition, no statistically significant differences in skin epithelium (U = 12.0, p = 0.911), blood vessels (U = 10.5, p = 0.661), sweat gland ducts (U = 0, p = 0.180), adipose glands (U = 1.5, p = 0.374), and hair follicles (U = 4.5, p = 0.297) were found (Table 12).

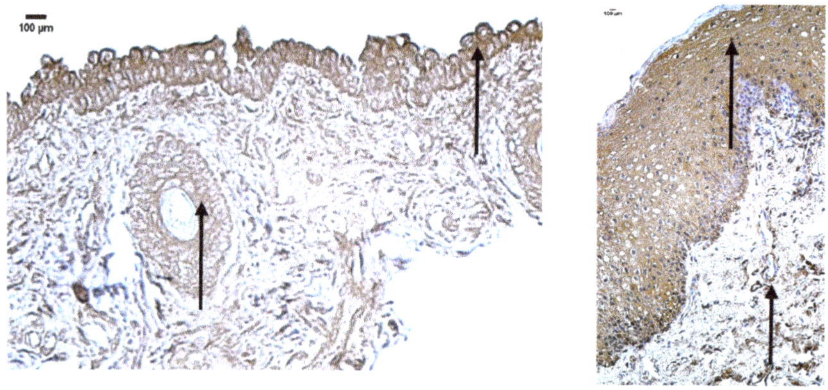

(**a**) (**b**)

Figure 10. Immunohistochemistry of the IL-10-positive structures in the control and patient tissue samples: (**a**) control sample with rare occurrence of IL-10-positive structures in adipose glands, few in mucosal epithelium and blood vessels, moderate in skin epithelium, hair follicles, and connective tissue (arrows), 200×; (**b**) patient sample with few IL-10-positive structures in skin epithelium, few to moderate in connective tissue, moderate in blood vessels and hair follicles, numerous in mucosal epithelium and sweat gland ducts (arrows), 200×.

3.10. Comparison of Defense Factor Appearance and Distribution

A visual summary of the comparison between immunity defense factor median values in the patient group and control group tissue samples is illustrated in Figure 11, where the overall differences between CD163, IL4, and the HBDs' distribution across the tissues can be seen.

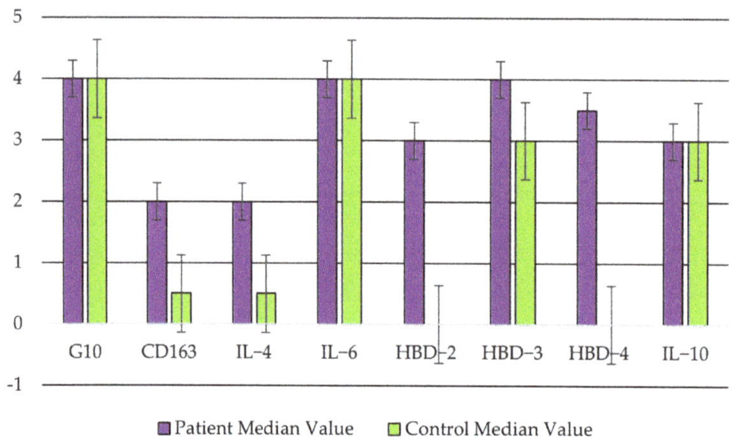

Median number	Explanation
0	0
1	0/+
2	+
3	+/++
4	++
5	++/+++
6	+++
7	+++/++++
8	++++

Figure 11. Comparison of immunity defense factor median distribution in patient and control group tissues.

3.11. Correlation in the Epithelium and Structures of Connective Tissue of Patient Group

Using Spearman's rank correlation coefficient, multiple statistically significant correlations ($p < 0.005$) were obtained between the factors in epithelium and connective tissue structures (Figures 12 and 13). The factors presented both positive (red) and negative (blue) correlations, with the biggest amount of statistically notable correlations being present in the epithelium of the patient tissue samples.

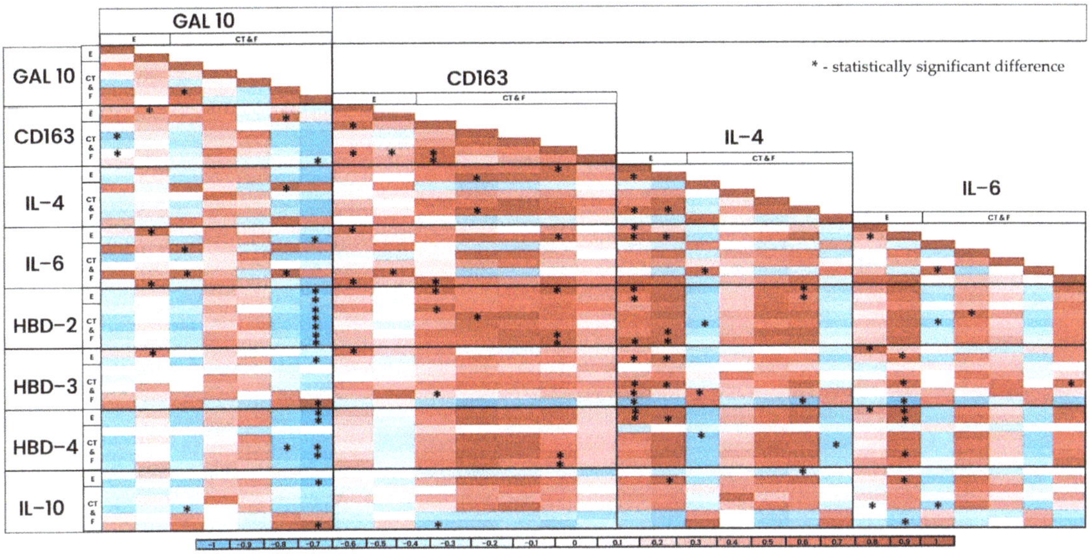

Figure 12. Heat-map of correlations between the factors (part one).

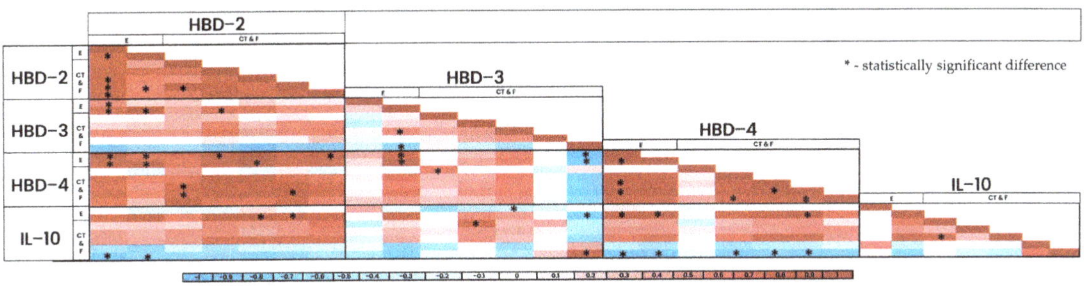

Figure 13. Heat-map of correlations between the factors (part two).

4. Discussion

In our study, a statistically significant increase in HBD-2-, HBD-3-, and HBD-4-positive structures was found in skin and the mucosal epithelium, hair follicles, and blood vessels of patient samples. A notable increase was also seen in IL-4, IL-6, and IL-10 in the mucosal epithelium and CD163 in the blood vessels. The connective tissue of patient samples presented with statistically significant decreases in Gal-10, IL-10, and HBD-3.

CD-163 is known to be a specific and important marker for M2 anti-inflammatory macrophages and their alternative activation [11,13]. Due to the alternative activation path of M2 macrophages, they present as anti-inflammatory by increasing tissue repair, angiogenesis, and expressing anti-inflammatory markers and cytokines like IL-10 [13,60]. It is also well-known that macrophages, especially M2 macrophages, play a crucial role in the event of vascular injury by recovering blood flow, repairing the vessel, resolving inflammation, and promoting wound healing [61]. These angiogenetic functions are ensured by the enhancement of endothelial cell proliferation, migration, and interactions with PFGFBB, MMP, TGFB1, and VEGF [62]. In our study, CD-163 significantly increased around the blood vessels of the patient group; therefore, this leads to a possible suggestion that in bilateral cleft lip and palate, the M1/M2 macrophage equilibrium is possibly shifted toward M2 macrophages to ensure angiogenesis and, therefore, resolution of chronic inflammation and better tissue healing in order to regain tissue homeostasis.

Human beta-defensins are antimicrobial peptides that control the process of inflammation or infection by the elimination of pathogens, improvement of wound healing, as well as by controlling cell proliferation, migration, chemotaxis, and cytokine production [40–43]. They form the first line of defense of epithelial tissues that ensure immune response and homeostasis [38,39,44]. Changes in HBD levels suggest impaired functions of the epithelial and mucosal barrier and increased susceptibility of pathogen invasion and infection development [37,43,63]. They are most commonly secreted by epithelial cells, therefore, they are most prominent in the structure of the epithelium, as well as the salivary glands [37,40,64]. The main upregulating factor for HBD secretion is inflammation or infection; hence, the upregulation of human beta-defensins in skin epithelium, mucosal epithelium, hair follicles, and blood vessels indicate the presence of chronic inflammation, as well as the presence of a line of defense that tries to regain tissue homeostasis of cleft-affected tissue [37–39,44] and characterizes also our patient bilateral cleft-affected lips.

An increase in HBD-4 expression in the skin and mucosal epithelium and increase in HBD-3 expression in mucosal epithelium mostly indicates the antimicrobial effects via the formation of pores in the cell membranes of pathogenic microorganisms [37], and an increase in mast cell degranulation, chemotaxis, and cytokine production [41,48–50]. The increase in HBD-2 secretion in the skin and mucosal epithelium, blood vessels, and hair follicles as well as the increase in HBD-3 secretion suggests that the overexpression of these factors severely increases healing to overcompensate the damage of tissue that has been caused by the chronic inflammation and restore normal protective functions of the epithelial barrier [41]. Furthermore, in our study, a significant decrease in HBD-3 was observed in the connective tissue of the patient group, which suggests impaired protection against pathogens and increased susceptibility to infections [37,43,63]. The inversed expression of HBD-3 in connective tissue and mucosal epithelium can possibly be explained by the fact that due to the nature of the cleft lip defect, the factor is significantly more necessary in the epithelium where the defect is the most severe; therefore, the overexpression in the epithelium is balanced by under-expression in the underlying connective tissue.

IL-4 is an anti-inflammatory cytokine that reduces inflammation, maintains homeostasis, promotes tissue repair, and decreases the release of pro-inflammatory cytokines [15,17,19,65,66]. It is one of the first and most important modulators that start the Th2 immune response (allergy, parasites) by instigating the cascade of CD4+ T cell, Th2 cell, B cell, and plasma cell differentiation, IgE secretion, and macrophage accumulation [67,68]. In our study, IL-4 levels in the mucosal epithelium were increased, therefore, it can be suggested that IL-4 functions as a protective agent that prevents excessive damage of the tissue that can be caused by the organism's immune response and the state of chronic inflammation [18]. Interestingly, when looking at functions of IL-4 in the epithelium and more specifically in keratinocytes, a healing-impairing function has been noted in a study conducted by Serezani et al. [69]. This effect could possibly be explained by the fact that with the decrease in healing properties in the mucosal epithelium, the overexpression of IL-4 ensures that the environment is suitable for the development of chronic infections.

IL-6 is a regulatory inflammatory cytokine that is secreted as a defense mechanism to tissue infections and injuries [23–26]. Increased levels of IL-6 promote active effects of the immune system via B- and T-cell differentiation, Ig secretion, ACP synthesis, and cell apoptosis [19,24]. However, decreased levels of IL-6 are important in the end stages of an immune reaction to ensure reparative functions and wound closure [70]. IL-6 has also been mentioned as an important promoter of chronic inflammation via regulation of T-cell differentiation [25,71]. Therefore, the increased expression of IL-6 in our study suggests that overexpression of IL-6 in the mucosal epithelium has a similar effect to the increase in IL-4—the factor promotes the state of inflammation and immune reaction, decreases the opportunity for the tissue to heal and, therefore, makes the tissue environment more suitable for chronic infections.

IL-10 also presents with anti-inflammatory effects by inhibiting pro-inflammatory cytokine secretion, antigen presentation, maintaining tissue homeostasis, and preventing tissue damage, all with the objective to resolve inflammation [28,30,72–74]. In Th1 cells, IL-10 ensures that the Th1 immune response is not excessive and destructive, and IL-10 from Th2 cells suppresses Th1 cells; however, in macrophages, it ensures the formation of a self-regulating macrophage population [28,31,75]. These functions that differ through cell types ensure that the immune response is regulated through all stages via different signaling pathways [29,30,76]. Due to IL-10′s anti-inflammatory nature, it is critical to carefully regulate and monitor its secretion to avoid excessive immunosuppression or immune activity [75]. In this study, the quantity of IL-10 was increased in mucosal epithelium, hence, the upregulation of this interleukin once again presents with the same effect and continues to add to the suppression of excessive inflammation and the creation of a favorable environment for prolonged infections [29,30]. Therefore, all three interleukins that were observed in this study create a high-functioning cascade that tries to increase healing and wound repair via different pathways; however, the effect that is created is more negative and makes the already infected and inflamed clefted tissue more suitable for the continuance of infections, immune responses, and tissue destruction.

Moreover, when looking at the connective tissue of the patient group, the IL-10 quantity was decreased. IL-10 is fundamental in the healing, wound repair, and scar formation process due to the fact that it increases epitheliocyte proliferation, hyaluronan synthesis, TGF- β expression, and induces ECM remodeling [73]. It has also been noted that IL-10 promotes the correct organization of collagen fibers during wound formation [35]. For these reasons, it can be suggested that the decrease in IL-10 observed in our study points to disrupted healing of the connective tissue and excessive scarring and fibrosis of the damaged area; therefore, making it more difficult for the clefted lip to heal properly and to be successfully repaired without compromising any functional or aesthetic parameters.

Gal-10 is a protein mainly found in human eosinophils, which is released into the tissue during eosinophil extracellular trap cell death [5,6,77,78]. The main functions of this protein are connected to immune responses targeted to parasites or allergic substances, inflammatory cytokine, chemokine, and prostaglandin release, as well as to participate in the EETosis, which ensnares and kills the pathogenic microorganisms that have entered the body [5,6,8,77,79,80]. Based on this information, the decrease in Gal-10 in the connective tissue of the patient group points to decreased eosinophilic function which, therefore, makes the tissue more susceptible to pathogenic, allergic, and parasitic infections as well as eosinophilic inflammation [5,7,77]. In a study performed by Buschmann et al., the increased levels of Gal-10 were connected to the development and maintenance of chronic inflammation [5]. For this reason, the decrease observed in this study could also be explained as a protective mechanism, where the cells of the connective tissue are attempting to decrease the presence of inflammation, which is promoted by various other local tissue factors. It is also important to note that Gal-10 has been previously connected to various pathologies connected to the nasal region, therefore, the change in this factor in the case of bilateral cleft lip could also point to the pathophysiological connection between the lip and nose in the case of this orofacial defect.

When looking at statistically significant correlations, multiple positive and negative correlations were observed between all of the factors in various tissue locations—skin and mucosal epithelium, blood vessels, sweat and adipose glands, hair follicles, and connective tissue. Correlations do not always mean causality; therefore, the interpretation of these results cannot always indicate the formation of a meaningful link between the factors. However, the possible connections of the synergistic actions of these factors are described as follows:

Galectin-10:

1. CD-163. Several positive correlations were observed between Gal-10 and CD-163. Gal-10 is characterized by its eosinophilic functions, eosinophilic inflammation, and release during EETosis [5,6,78], mostly with a destructive nature. On the other hand, CD163 is connected to M2 macrophages, which are characterized by their anti-inflammatory nature, improvement of healing, and downregulation of inflammation [12,14]. In

a study conducted by Liu et al., it was noted that in various bacterial and parasite infections, M2 macrophages protect the body from excessive tissue damage by clearing apoptotic cells and inducing regeneration [81]; hence, connecting the functions of these two factors, it can be suggested that this positive correlation between them indicates mutual synergy, where Gal-10 creates tissue inflammation to protect it from invaders but M2 macrophages work alongside it to clear the created debris and to preserve the tissue from extreme inflammatory damage;

2. IL-6. Mostly positive correlations in the epithelial parts of the samples, which point to a mutual increase in inflammatory reactions;
3. IL-4. One positive correlation between IL-4 and Gal-10 was observed, which can be explained by the similar secretion mechanisms of both factors—either can be secreted by eosionphils, basophils, or T cells [5,6,15–17,67,68,77];
4. HBD-2, -3, and -4. Mostly negative correlations and only in the connective tissue were observed between the human beta-defensins and galectin-10. This could mean that the increased activity of Gal-10 and eosinophilic functions suppress the antimicrobial and healing properties of human beta-defensins, creating an environment more suitable for developing and sustaining chronic inflammation;
5. IL-10. Similarly, correlations dominate in the connective tissue and are mostly negative, which continues the link of increased inflammation via Gal-10 activation and the suppression of healing and restorative properties through a decrease in anti-inflammatory IL-10.

CD-163:

1. IL-4. In order for macrophages to polarize into the M2 subtype, they have to go through an alternative activation path during the inflammatory response with IL-1, IL-4, IL-6, IL-13, TGF-β, TLR, and glucocorticoids [11,13]. Polarization of the macrophages into M1 (killer) or M2 (healer) phenotypes creates a delicate equilibrium between pro- and anti-inflammatory occurrences in the body and ensures balance between inflammation and its resolution [60,82]. Some positive correlations were noted between IL-4 and CD-163 in the epithelium and connective tissue, which can be explained by the fact that macrophage polarization into the M2 subtype—which expresses CD-163—is carried out through an alternative activation path during the inflammatory response with IL-4 as a mediating agent [11,13]. Previously, possible connections between IL-4 and M2 macrophages and tissue healing have been suggested [83];
2. IL-6. Similarly, positive correlations were observed with IL-6 because IL-6 also increases M2 macrophage polarization and CD-163 expression [11–13,84]. Moreover, M2 macrophages have been noted to induce IL-6 secretion [12,14];
3. IL-10. One negative correlation in the connective tissue was seen. This finding is contrary to previous studies, where IL-10 was noted to induce M2 polarization [85] and where M2 macrophages secreted IL-10 [12,14]. IL-10 has also been noted to maintain tissue homeostasis and resolve inflammation with inhibiting antigen presentation to macrophages [28,30,72–74]. Therefore, the finding of our study could point to the suppression of IL-10 with the aim of maintaining antigen presentation and active functions of M2 macrophages;
4. HBD-2, -3, and -4. Several positive correlations were noted, which can be explained by the similar functions of these factors—all of them can improve healing, angiogenesis, antimicrobial effects, and inflammation resolution [12,14,40–43].

IL-4:

1. IL-6. Several positive correlations were noted between the factors. In previous studies, in order for the tissue and wound to heal properly and without any complications, it had been noted that IL-6 and IL-4 levels change inversely—during the healing stages IL-6 decreases but IL-4 increases to facilitate wound repair and M2 activity [70,86,87]. Therefore, the results of this study are contrary as they suggest that in the case of

cleft lip, the mechanism of normal wound healing is impaired and the patient is more susceptible to infections, fibrosis, scarring, and hypertrophic scar formation [70];

2. IL-10. One positive correlation in the epithelium was observed between IL-4 and L-10. Both of these factors are mentioned to promote tissue repair, reduce inflammation, maintain homeostasis, and suppress excessive inflammation [28]. Moreover, a possible link between these factors has been previously noted as well as the fact that IL-10 can be upregulated by IL-4 [28,33,83]. For these reasons, it is clear that IL-10 and IL-4 both function synergistically to fight the extensive inflammation that is characteristic of cleft-affected tissue;
3. HBD-2, -3, and -4. A vast amount of positive correlations were observed between HBD-2, -3, and -4 and some negative correlations were also present between IL-4 and HBD-4. The positive correlations can also be explained by the similar anti-inflammatory functions of the factors but the negative correlation between IL-4 and HBD-4 could suggest impairment of the epithelial barrier and its protective functions [48].

IL-6:

1. IL-10. Mostly negative correlations were observed, which are in accordance with previous studies—where, during the tissue-healing phase, IL-6 decreases and IL-10 increases to facilitate successful wound repair [86,87]. However, some studies have also shown directly increasing links between IL-6 and IL-10, mostly in cases of chronically driven inflammation where prominent tissue degeneration is present [27, 86–89]. Therefore, it can be assumed that in the tissues of cleft lip, IL-6 and IL-10 are cooperating in a manner of maximal healing induction to promote faster and more adequate wound repair;
2. HBD-2, -3, and -4. Mostly positive correlations were observed between IL-6 and all of the human beta-defensins, which suggest that human beta-defensins and IL-6 mutually stimulate one another to facilitate and drive the inflammation toward the desired resolution of the process [39–41,48–50].

HBDs:

3. IL-10. Both positive and negative correlations were observed between IL-10 and HBD-2, -3, and -4. The positive correlations can be explained by the anti-inflammatory mutual stimulation and induction of the factors to ensure more prominent healing, repairing, and homeostatic effects [39,40]. In addition, the negative correlations could point to IL-10′s downregulating effects on the HBD's pro-inflammatory effects, like antimicrobial action and induction of immune and inflammatory reactions [90];
4. HBDs. All of the human beta-defensins were mutually positively correlated in the epithelium and connective tissues of the samples, which continues to suggest the similar functions of all these antimicrobial peptides and their link with one another in order to induce the most effective and comprehensive protective effects for the cleft-affected lip tissue. However, there was also a negative correlation between HBD-3 and HBD-4, which is contrary to previous studies—where a strong link between HBD-3 and HBD-4 and their functions has been described [37,39]. This leads to believe that the cooperative effect between these factors that usually ensures comprehensive protection of epithelium, mucosa, and the underlying tissue is severely impaired in the case of cleft lip.

Moreover, when comparing the results of this study with results obtained in previous studies researching the same factors in cleft palate-affected patients of the same age group, it can be seen that in the case of the cleft lip, local tissue defense factors present with more notable increases in their levels but in cleft palate they were mostly decreased [91]. This phenomenon can be explained by the fact that cleft lip is a defect that is morphologically and clinically more connected to the outer environment; therefore, it should present with more prominent inflammatory and immunological processes. The deviance that was consistent in both of these studies is the decrease in HBD-3 in connective tissue, which continues to prove the significance of HBD-3 in cleft defects and its role in the suppression of connective tissue healing and homeostasis. In both studies, the correlations between HBDs were also similar, which continues to be a reliable proof of the changes in the epithelial barriers and healing properties of cleft-affected tissues.

It is also noteworthy to mention that the connections between clefted tissue and local tissue defense factors observed in this study are novel findings due to the severity of the defect that is present in patients with bilateral cleft lip. Bilateral cleft lip is the most severe form of cleft, therefore, the patient presents with a distinct scarcity of tissue material. This results in not only more technically difficult surgery but also in almost impossible acquisition of excess tissue material for scientific samples. Moreover, the novelty of this study is further extended with the young age of the patients and scarcity of other studies researching this specific age group (until the age of milk dentition).

A noteworthy limitation of our study could be the inconsistent presence of all tissue structures in the patient tissue samples—some lacked hair follicles, adipose glands, sweat glands, or some parts of the epithelium. This limitation is closely connected to the severity of the bilateral cleft lip defect and scarcity of the tissue material present. The main causal factor for this limitation is the fact that the tissue samples can only be acquired when they are not needed for the sufficient repair of the clefted defect during cheiloplasty surgery. Due to the reason that the patients are young and small, the amount of tissue necessary for the reconstruction is already scarce, so any additional and unneeded tissue material is rarely present in these cases. Moreover, the tissue pieces that can be used for scientific sample acquisition will not always be identical and with the same tissue structures present because all of the best parts of the tissue have been used for the patient reconstruction, and every case of BCLP and its reconstruction is different and requires different approaches to close the defect with only using the available tissue present. For this reason, the tissue that is left will always be different and sometimes may even be damaged during the reconstructive process, therefore, missing certain tissue structures.

Moreover, to gain a clearer insight about the defense factor concentration and gene distribution, other methods like ELISA and in situ hybridization could be used as well as longitudinal correlations between the changes in the factors and clinical state of the patients throughout the years and many follow-up surgeries.

5. Conclusions

Generally, in BCLP tissues, an increase in HBDs, M2 macrophages, IL-4, and IL-6, was observed, while IL-10 and Gal-10 showed a significant decrease.

The increase in ILs and HBDs suggests increased healing and wound repair, which is complemented by chronic inflammation and a larger susceptibility to chronic and continuous infections.

An attempt to reduce the presence of inflammation could be explained by the decrease in IL-10 and Gal-10, which points to compromised and fibrotic tissue healing as well as decreased eosinophilic functions.

The increase in CD163 around the blood vessels could signal a possible shift in the M1/M2 macrophage equilibrium toward M2 macrophages to ensure angiogenesis, resolution of inflammation, and tissue healing.

The presence of various positive and negative mutual correlations between the factors indicates mutually linked effects, especially between HBDs and ILs, which function as important and synergistic mediators of immunological, inflammatory, and homeostatic processes that occur in the tissues of bilateral cleft lip.

Author Contributions: Conceptualization, M.P.; methodology, M.P.; software, L.O.; validation, M.P.; formal analysis, L.O.; investigation, M.P.; resources, M.P.; data curation, M.P.; writing—original draft preparation, L.O.; writing—review and editing, M.P. and L.O.; visualization, L.O.; supervision, M.P.; project administration, M.P.; funding acquisition, M.P. All authors have read and agreed to the published version of the manuscript.

Funding: This research received no external funding.

Institutional Review Board Statement: This study was conducted in accordance with the Declaration of Helsinki and approved by the Ethics Committee of Riga Stradins University (22 May 2003; 17 January 2013; 5/25 June 2018; Nr. 2-PEK-4/595/2022).

Informed Consent Statement: Informed consent was obtained from all subjects involved in this study.

Data Availability Statement: All datasets used in the present study are available in Section 3.

Acknowledgments: We would like to express our gratitude to Ilze Akota of the Institute of Stomatology at RSU for contributing the patient material as well as to Laboratory Assistant Natalija Moroza for processing and preparing the tissue material. Additionally, we would like to acknowledge the patients' parents for their willingness to take part in the present study. Rīga Stradinš University's kind support for the research is also highly acknowledged.

Conflicts of Interest: The authors declare no conflicts of interest.

References

1. Alois, C.I.; Ruotolo, R.A. An overview of cleft lip and palate. *Jaapa* **2020**, *33*, 17–20. [CrossRef]
2. Hattori, Y.; Pai, B.C.; Saito, T.; Chou, P.Y.; Lu, T.C.; Chang, C.S.; Chen, Y.R.; Lo, L.J. Long-term treatment outcome of patients with complete bilateral cleft lip and palate: A retrospective cohort study. *Int. J. Surg.* **2023**, *109*, 1656–1667. [CrossRef]
3. Costa, B.; Lima, J.E.; Gomide, M.R.; Rosa, O.P. Clinical and microbiological evaluation of the periodontal status of children with unilateral complete cleft lip and palate. *Cleft Palate Craniofac. J.* **2003**, *40*, 585–589. [CrossRef]
4. Dings, R.P.M.; Miller, M.C.; Griffin, R.J.; Mayo, K.H. Galectins as Molecular Targets for Therapeutic Intervention. *Int. J. Mol. Sci.* **2018**, *19*, 905. [CrossRef]
5. Buschmann, C.; Unverdorben, L.; Knabl, J.; Hutter, S.; Meister, S.; Beyer, S.; Burgmann, M.; Keilmann, L.; Zati Zehni, A.; Schmoeckel, E.; et al. Galectin-10 Expression in Placentas of Women with Gestational Diabetes. *Curr. Issues Mol. Biol.* **2023**, *45*, 8840–8851. [CrossRef]
6. Fukuchi, M.; Kamide, Y.; Ueki, S.; Miyabe, Y.; Konno, Y.; Oka, N.; Takeuchi, H.; Koyota, S.; Hirokawa, M.; Yamada, T.; et al. Eosinophil ETosis-Mediated Release of Galectin-10 in Eosinophilic Granulomatosis with Polyangiitis. *Arthritis Rheumatol.* **2021**, *73*, 1683–1693. [CrossRef]
7. Kwarteng, A.; Mensah, C.; Osei-Poku, P. Eosinophil: An innate immune cell with anti-filarial vaccine and biomarker potential. *Health Sci. Rep.* **2023**, *6*, e1320. [CrossRef]
8. Kim, J.S.; Cho, I.H.; Kim, K.H.; Hwang, Y.S. Identification of galectin-10 as a biomarker for periodontitis based on proteomic analysis of gingival crevicular fluid. *Mol. Med. Rep.* **2021**, *23*, 123. [CrossRef]
9. Larsson, H.; Albinsson Högberg, S.; Lind, M.; Rabe, H.; Lingblom, C. Investigating immune profile by CyTOF in individuals with long-standing type 1 diabetes. *Sci. Rep.* **2023**, *13*, 8171. [CrossRef]
10. Etzerodt, A.; Moestrup, S.K. CD163 and inflammation: Biological, diagnostic, and therapeutic aspects. *Antioxid. Redox Signal.* **2013**, *18*, 2352–2363. [CrossRef]
11. Yap, Y.J.; Wong, P.F.; AbuBakar, S.; Sam, S.S.; Shunmugarajoo, A.; Soh, Y.H.; Misbah, S.; Ab Rahman, A.K. The clinical utility of CD163 in viral diseases. *Clin. Chim. Acta* **2023**, *541*, 117243. [CrossRef]
12. Van Gorp, H.; Delputte, P.L.; Nauwynck, H.J. Scavenger receptor CD163, a Jack-of-all-trades and potential target for cell-directed therapy. *Mol. Immunol.* **2010**, *47*, 1650–1660. [CrossRef]
13. Skytthe, M.K.; Graversen, J.H.; Moestrup, S.K. Targeting of CD163(+) Macrophages in Inflammatory and Malignant Diseases. *Int. J. Mol. Sci.* **2020**, *21*, 5497. [CrossRef]
14. Fabriek, B.O.; Dijkstra, C.D.; van den Berg, T.K. The macrophage scavenger receptor CD163. *Immunobiology* **2005**, *210*, 153–160. [CrossRef]
15. Lima Teixeira, J.F.; Henning, P.; Cintra Magalhães, F.A.; Coletto-Nunes, G.; Floriano-Marcelino, T.; Westerlund, A.; Movérare-Skrtic, S.; Oliveira, G.; Lerner, U.H.; Souza, P.P.C. Osteoprotective effect by interleukin-4 (IL-4) on lipoprotein-induced periodontitis. *Cytokine* **2023**, *172*, 156399. [CrossRef]
16. Ujiie, Y.; Karakida, T.; Yamakoshi, Y.; Ohshima, T.; Gomi, K.; Oida, S. Interleukin-4 released from human gingival fibroblasts reduces osteoclastogenesis. *Arch. Oral. Biol.* **2016**, *72*, 187–193. [CrossRef]
17. Tognarelli, E.I.; Gutiérrez-Vera, C.; Palacios, P.A.; Pasten-Ferrada, I.A.; Aguirre-Muñoz, F.; Cornejo, D.A.; González, P.A.; Carreño, L.J. Natural Killer T Cell Diversity and Immunotherapy. *Cancers* **2023**, *15*, 5737. [CrossRef]
18. Chmielecki, A.; Bortnik, K.; Galczynski, S.; Kopacz, K.; Padula, G.; Jerczynska, H.; Stawski, R.; Nowak, D. Interleukin-4 during post-exercise recovery negatively correlates with the production of phagocyte-generated oxidants. *Front. Physiol.* **2023**, *14*, 1186296. [CrossRef]
19. Pilmane, M.; Sidhoma, E.; Akota, I.; Kazoka, D. Characterization of Cytokines and Proliferation Marker Ki67 in Cleft Affected Lip Tissue. *Medicina* **2019**, *55*, 518. [CrossRef]
20. Gould, S.J.; Foey, A.D.; Salih, V.M. An organotypic oral mucosal infection model to study host-pathogen interactions. *J. Tissue Eng.* **2023**, *14*, 20417314231197310. [CrossRef]

21. Muñoz-Cánoves, P.; Scheele, C.; Pedersen, B.K.; Serrano, A.L. Interleukin-6 myokine signaling in skeletal muscle: A double-edged sword? *FEBS J.* **2013**, *280*, 4131–4148. [CrossRef] [PubMed]
22. Jordan, S.C.; Ammerman, N.; Huang, E.; Vo, A. Importance of IL-6 inhibition in prevention and treatment of antibody-mediated rejection in kidney allografts. *Am. J. Transplant.* **2022**, *22* (Suppl. 4), 28–37. [CrossRef] [PubMed]
23. Toprak, V.; Akalın, S.A.; Öcal, E.; Çavuş, Y.; Deveci, E. Biochemical and immunohistochemical examination of the effects of ephedrine in rat ovary tissue. *Acta Cir. Bras.* **2023**, *38*, e381523. [CrossRef] [PubMed]
24. Elner, V.M.; Scales, W.; Elner, S.G.; Danforth, J.; Kunkel, S.L.; Strieter, R.M. Interleukin-6 (IL-6) gene expression and secretion by cytokine-stimulated human retinal pigment epithelial cells. *Exp. Eye Res.* **1992**, *54*, 361–368. [CrossRef]
25. Tanaka, T.; Narazaki, M.; Kishimoto, T. IL-6 in inflammation, immunity, and disease. *Cold Spring Harb. Perspect. Biol.* **2014**, *6*, a016295. [CrossRef]
26. Benson, M.T.; Shepherd, L.; Rees, R.C.; Rennie, I.G. Production of interleukin-6 by human retinal pigment epithelium in vitro and its regulation by other cytokines. *Curr. Eye Res.* **1992**, *11* (Suppl. 1), 173–179. [CrossRef] [PubMed]
27. Roy, A.; Ben Lagha, A.; Gonçalves, R.; Grenier, D. Effects of Saliva from Periodontally Healthy and Diseased Subjects on Barrier Function and the Inflammatory Response in in vitro Models of the Oral Epithelium. *Front. Oral. Health* **2021**, *2*, 815728. [CrossRef]
28. Ouyang, W.; Rutz, S.; Crellin, N.K.; Valdez, P.A.; Hymowitz, S.G. Regulation and functions of the IL-10 family of cytokines in inflammation and disease. *Annu. Rev. Immunol.* **2011**, *29*, 71–109. [CrossRef]
29. Ouyang, W.; O'Garra, A. IL-10 Family Cytokines IL-10 and IL-22: From Basic Science to Clinical Translation. *Immunity* **2019**, *50*, 871–891. [CrossRef]
30. Carlini, V.; Noonan, D.M.; Abdalalem, E.; Goletti, D.; Sansone, C.; Calabrone, L.; Albini, A. The multifaceted nature of IL-10: Regulation, role in immunological homeostasis and its relevance to cancer, COVID-19 and post-COVID conditions. *Front. Immunol.* **2023**, *14*, 1161067. [CrossRef]
31. Wei, H.X.; Wang, B.; Li, B. IL-10 and IL-22 in Mucosal Immunity: Driving Protection and Pathology. *Front. Immunol.* **2020**, *11*, 1315. [CrossRef]
32. Wei, Z.; Su, X.; Hu, Q.; Huang, Y.; Li, C.; Huang, X. Association of interleukin-10 rs1800896, rs1800872, and interleukin-6 rs1800795 polymorphisms with squamous cell carcinoma risk: A meta-analysis. *Open Life Sci.* **2023**, *18*, 20220580. [CrossRef]
33. Hazlett, L.D.; Jiang, X.; McClellan, S.A. IL-10 function, regulation, and in bacterial keratitis. *J. Ocul. Pharmacol. Ther.* **2014**, *30*, 373–380. [CrossRef]
34. Geginat, J.; Vasco, M.; Gerosa, M.; Tas, S.W.; Pagani, M.; Grassi, F.; Flavell, R.A.; Meroni, P.; Abrignani, S. IL-10 producing regulatory and helper T-cells in systemic lupus erythematosus. *Semin. Immunol.* **2019**, *44*, 101330. [CrossRef]
35. Peranteau, W.H.; Zhang, L.; Muvarak, N.; Badillo, A.T.; Radu, A.; Zoltick, P.W.; Liechty, K.W. IL-10 overexpression decreases inflammatory mediators and promotes regenerative healing in an adult model of scar formation. *J. Investig. Dermatol.* **2008**, *128*, 1852–1860. [CrossRef]
36. Short, W.D.; Steen, E.; Kaul, A.; Wang, X.; Olutoye, O.O., 2nd; Vangapandu, H.V.; Templeman, N.; Blum, A.J.; Moles, C.M.; Narmoneva, D.A.; et al. IL-10 promotes endothelial progenitor cell infiltration and wound healing via STAT3. *FASEB J.* **2022**, *36*, e22298. [CrossRef]
37. Yanagi, S.; Ashitani, J.; Ishimoto, H.; Date, Y.; Mukae, H.; Chino, N.; Nakazato, M. Isolation of human beta-defensin-4 in lung tissue and its increase in lower respiratory tract infection. *Respir. Res.* **2005**, *6*, 130. [CrossRef]
38. Paris, S.; Wolgin, M.; Kielbassa, A.M.; Pries, A.; Zakrzewicz, A. Gene expression of human beta-defensins in healthy and inflamed human dental pulps. *J. Endod.* **2009**, *35*, 520–523. [CrossRef]
39. Chen, X.; Niyonsaba, F.; Ushio, H.; Hara, M.; Yokoi, H.; Matsumoto, K.; Saito, H.; Nagaoka, I.; Ikeda, S.; Okumura, K.; et al. Antimicrobial peptides human beta-defensin (hBD)-3 and hBD-4 activate mast cells and increase skin vascular permeability. *Eur. J. Immunol.* **2007**, *37*, 434–444. [CrossRef]
40. Li, X.; Duan, D.; Yang, J.; Wang, P.; Han, B.; Zhao, L.; Jepsen, S.; Dommisch, H.; Winter, J.; Xu, Y. The expression of human β-defensins (hBD-1, hBD-2, hBD-3, hBD-4) in gingival epithelia. *Arch. Oral. Biol.* **2016**, *66*, 15–21. [CrossRef]
41. Hirsch, T.; Spielmann, M.; Zuhaili, B.; Fossum, M.; Metzig, M.; Koehler, T.; Steinau, H.U.; Yao, F.; Onderdonk, A.B.; Steinstraesser, L.; et al. Human beta-defensin-3 promotes wound healing in infected diabetic wounds. *J. Gene Med.* **2009**, *11*, 220–228. [CrossRef]
42. Supp, D.M.; Karpinski, A.C.; Boyce, S.T. Expression of human beta-defensins HBD-1, HBD-2, and HBD-3 in cultured keratinocytes and skin substitutes. *Burns* **2004**, *30*, 643–648. [CrossRef]
43. Mi, B.; Liu, J.; Liu, Y.; Hu, L.; Panayi, A.C.; Zhou, W.; Liu, G. The Designer Antimicrobial Peptide A-hBD-2 Facilitates Skin Wound Healing by Stimulating Keratinocyte Migration and Proliferation. *Cell Physiol. Biochem.* **2018**, *51*, 647–663. [CrossRef]
44. Pereira, A.L.; Franco, G.C.; Cortelli, S.C.; Aquino, D.R.; Costa, F.O.; Raslan, S.A.; Cortelli, J.R. Influence of periodontal status and periodontopathogens on levels of oral human β-defensin-2 in saliva. *J. Periodontol.* **2013**, *84*, 1445–1453. [CrossRef]
45. Schittek, B. The antimicrobial skin barrier in patients with atopic dermatitis. *Curr. Probl. Dermatol.* **2011**, *41*, 54–67. [CrossRef]
46. Varoga, D.; Klostermeier, E.; Paulsen, F.; Wruck, C.; Lippross, S.; Brandenburg, L.O.; Tohidnezhad, M.; Seekamp, A.; Tillmann, B.; Pufe, T. The antimicrobial peptide HBD-2 and the Toll-like receptors-2 and -4 are induced in synovial membranes in case of septic arthritis. *Virchows Arch.* **2009**, *454*, 685–694. [CrossRef]
47. Dommisch, H.; Staufenbiel, I.; Schulze, K.; Stiesch, M.; Winkel, A.; Fimmers, R.; Dommisch, J.; Jepsen, S.; Miosge, N.; Adam, K.; et al. Expression of antimicrobial peptides and interleukin-8 during early stages of inflammation: An experimental gingivitis study. *J. Periodontal Res.* **2015**, *50*, 836–845. [CrossRef]

48. Peng, G.; Tsukamoto, S.; Ikutama, R.; Nguyen, H.L.T.; Umehara, Y.; Trujillo-Paez, J.V.; Yue, H.; Takahashi, M.; Ogawa, T.; Kishi, R.; et al. Human β-defensin-3 attenuates atopic dermatitis-like inflammation through autophagy activation and the aryl hydrocarbon receptor signaling pathway. *J. Clin. Investig.* **2022**, *132*, e156501. [CrossRef]
49. Judge, C.J.; Reyes-Aviles, E.; Conry, S.J.; Sieg, S.S.; Feng, Z.; Weinberg, A.; Anthony, D.D. HBD-3 induces NK cell activation, IFN-γ secretion and mDC dependent cytolytic function. *Cell Immunol.* **2015**, *297*, 61–68. [CrossRef]
50. Chessa, C.; Bodet, C.; Jousselin, C.; Larivière, A.; Damour, A.; Garnier, J.; Lévêque, N.; Garcia, M. Antiviral Effect of hBD-3 and LL-37 during Human Primary Keratinocyte Infection with West Nile Virus. *Viruses* **2022**, *14*, 1552. [CrossRef]
51. Schneider, J.J.; Unholzer, A.; Schaller, M.; Schäfer-Korting, M.; Korting, H.C. Human defensins. *J. Mol. Med.* **2005**, *83*, 587–595. [CrossRef]
52. Zhu, C.; Bao, N.R.; Chen, S.; Zhao, J.N. HBD-3 regulation of the immune response and the LPS/TLR4-mediated signaling pathway. *Exp. Ther. Med.* **2016**, *12*, 2150–2154. [CrossRef]
53. Scheid, R.C.; Weiss, G. *Woelfel's Dental Anatomy*; Wolters Kluwer/Lippincott Williams & Wilkins Health: Philadelphia, PA, USA, 2012.
54. Suvarna, S.K.; Layton, C.; Bancroft, J.D. *Bancroft's Theory and Practice of Histological Techniques*; Elsevier: New York, NY, USA, 2019.
55. Deņisova, A.; Pilmane, M.; Kažoka, D. Antimicrobial Peptides and Interleukins in Cleft Soft Palate. *Children* **2023**, *10*, 1162. [CrossRef]
56. Vaivads, M.; Akota, I.; Pilmane, M. Cleft Candidate Genes and Their Products in Human Unilateral Cleft Lip Tissue. *Diseases* **2021**, *9*, 26. [CrossRef]
57. Vitenberga, Z.; Pilmane, M.; Babjoniševa, A. The evaluation of inflammatory, anti-inflammatory and regulatory factors contributing to the pathogenesis of COPD in airways. *Pathol. Res. Pract.* **2019**, *215*, 97–105. [CrossRef]
58. Barton, B.; Peat, J. *Medical Statistics: A Guide to SPSS, Data Analysis and Critical Appraisal*; Wiley: New York, NY, USA, 2014.
59. Vaivads, M.; Akota, I.; Pilmane, M. Characterization of SHH, SOX3, WNT3A and WNT9B Proteins in Human Non-Syndromic Cleft Lip and Palate Tissue. *Dent. J.* **2023**, *11*, 151. [CrossRef]
60. Iglesias-Linares, A.; Hartsfield, J.K., Jr. Cellular and Molecular Pathways Leading to External Root Resorption. *J. Dent. Res.* **2017**, *96*, 145–152. [CrossRef]
61. Hong, H.; Tian, X.Y. The Role of Macrophages in Vascular Repair and Regeneration after Ischemic Injury. *Int. J. Mol. Sci.* **2020**, *21*, 6328. [CrossRef]
62. Graney, P.L.; Ben-Shaul, S.; Landau, S.; Bajpai, A.; Singh, B.; Eager, J.; Cohen, A.; Levenberg, S.; Spiller, K.L. Macrophages of diverse phenotypes drive vascularization of engineered tissues. *Sci. Adv.* **2020**, *6*, eaay6391. [CrossRef]
63. Otte, J.M.; Neumann, H.M.; Brand, S.; Schrader, H.; Schmidt, W.E.; Schmitz, F. Expression of beta-defensin 4 is increased in human gastritis. *Eur. J. Clin. Investig.* **2009**, *39*, 126–138. [CrossRef]
64. Wolgin, M.; Liodakis, S.; Pries, A.R.; Zakrzewicz, A.; Kielbassa, A.M. HBD-1 and hBD-2 expression in HaCaT keratinocytes stimulated with nicotine. *Arch. Oral. Biol.* **2012**, *57*, 814–819. [CrossRef] [PubMed]
65. Bendixen, A.C.; Shevde, N.K.; Dienger, K.M.; Willson, T.M.; Funk, C.D.; Pike, J.W. IL-4 inhibits osteoclast formation through a direct action on osteoclast precursors via peroxisome proliferator-activated receptor gamma 1. *Proc. Natl. Acad. Sci. USA* **2001**, *98*, 2443–2448. [CrossRef] [PubMed]
66. Viksne, R.J.; Sumeraga, G.; Pilmane, M. Characterization of Cytokines and Proliferation Marker Ki67 in Chronic Rhinosinusitis with Nasal Polyps: A Pilot Study. *Medicina* **2021**, *57*, 607. [CrossRef] [PubMed]
67. Karo-Atar, D.; Bitton, A.; Benhar, I.; Munitz, A. Therapeutic Targeting of the Interleukin-4/Interleukin-13 Signaling Pathway: In Allergy and Beyond. *BioDrugs* **2018**, *32*, 201–220. [CrossRef]
68. Maurelli, M.; Chiricozzi, A.; Peris, K.; Gisondi, P.; Girolomoni, G. Atopic Dermatitis in the Elderly Population. *Acta Derm. Venereol.* **2023**, *103*, adv13363. [CrossRef]
69. Serezani, A.P.M.; Bozdogan, G.; Sehra, S.; Walsh, D.; Krishnamurthy, P.; Sierra Potchanant, E.A.; Nalepa, G.; Goenka, S.; Turner, M.J.; Spandau, D.F.; et al. IL-4 impairs wound healing potential in the skin by repressing fibronectin expression. *J. Allergy Clin. Immunol.* **2017**, *139*, 142–151.e5. [CrossRef]
70. Johnson, B.Z.; Stevenson, A.W.; Prêle, C.M.; Fear, M.W.; Wood, F.M. The Role of IL-6 in Skin Fibrosis and Cutaneous Wound Healing. *Biomedicines* **2020**, *8*, 101. [CrossRef]
71. Al-Rasheed, M.; Ball, C.; Parthiban, S.; Ganapathy, K. Evaluation of protection and immunity induced by infectious bronchitis vaccines administered by oculonasal, spray or gel routes in commercial broiler chicks. *Vaccine* **2023**, *41*, 4508–4524. [CrossRef]
72. Stanic, B.; van de Veen, W.; Wirz, O.F.; Rückert, B.; Morita, H.; Söllner, S.; Akdis, C.A.; Akdis, M. IL-10-overexpressing B cells regulate innate and adaptive immune responses. *J. Allergy Clin. Immunol.* **2015**, *135*, 771–780.e8. [CrossRef]
73. Singampalli, K.L.; Balaji, S.; Wang, X.; Parikh, U.M.; Kaul, A.; Gilley, J.; Birla, R.K.; Bollyky, P.L.; Keswani, S.G. The Role of an IL-10/Hyaluronan Axis in Dermal Wound Healing. *Front. Cell Dev. Biol.* **2020**, *8*, 636. [CrossRef]
74. Sun, Z.L.; Feng, Y.; Zou, M.L.; Zhao, B.H.; Liu, S.Y.; Du, Y.; Yu, S.; Yang, M.L.; Wu, J.J.; Yuan, Z.D.; et al. Emerging Role of IL-10 in Hypertrophic Scars. *Front. Med.* **2020**, *7*, 438. [CrossRef] [PubMed]
75. Hutchins, A.P.; Diez, D.; Miranda-Saavedra, D. The IL-10/STAT3-mediated anti-inflammatory response: Recent developments and future challenges. *Brief. Funct. Genom.* **2013**, *12*, 489–498. [CrossRef] [PubMed]
76. Saraiva, M.; Vieira, P.; O'Garra, A. Biology and therapeutic potential of interleukin-10. *J. Exp. Med.* **2020**, *217*, e20190418. [CrossRef] [PubMed]

77. Tomizawa, H.; Yamada, Y.; Arima, M.; Miyabe, Y.; Fukuchi, M.; Hikichi, H.; Melo, R.C.N.; Yamada, T.; Ueki, S. Galectin-10 as a Potential Biomarker for Eosinophilic Diseases. *Biomolecules* **2022**, *12*, 1385. [CrossRef]
78. Sato, T.; Chiba, T.; Nakahara, T.; Watanabe, K.; Sakai, S.; Noguchi, N.; Noto, M.; Ueki, S.; Kono, M. Eosinophil-derived galectin-10 upregulates matrix metalloproteinase expression in bullous pemphigoid blisters. *J. Dermatol. Sci.* **2023**, *112*, 6–14. [CrossRef] [PubMed]
79. Heyndrickx, I.; Deswarte, K.; Verstraete, K.; Verschueren, K.H.G.; Smole, U.; Aegerter, H.; Dansercoer, A.; Hammad, H.; Savvides, S.N.; Lambrecht, B.N. Ym1 protein crystals promote type 2 immunity. *eLife* **2024**, *12*, RP90676. [CrossRef]
80. Guimarães-Costa, A.B.; Nascimento, M.T.; Wardini, A.B.; Pinto-da-Silva, L.H.; Saraiva, E.M. ETosis: A Microbicidal Mechanism beyond Cell Death. *J. Parasitol. Res.* **2012**, *2012*, 929743. [CrossRef]
81. Liu, Y.C.; Zou, X.B.; Chai, Y.F.; Yao, Y.M. Macrophage polarization in inflammatory diseases. *Int. J. Biol. Sci.* **2014**, *10*, 520–529. [CrossRef]
82. Guo, L.; Akahori, H.; Harari, E.; Smith, S.L.; Polavarapu, R.; Karmali, V.; Otsuka, F.; Gannon, R.L.; Braumann, R.E.; Dickinson, M.H.; et al. CD163+ macrophages promote angiogenesis and vascular permeability accompanied by inflammation in atherosclerosis. *J. Clin. Investig.* **2018**, *128*, 1106–1124. [CrossRef]
83. Nikovics, K.; Favier, A.L.; Rocher, M.; Mayinga, C.; Gomez, J.; Dufour-Gaume, F.; Riccobono, D. In Situ Identification of Both IL-4 and IL-10 Cytokine-Receptor Interactions during Tissue Regeneration. *Cells* **2023**, *12*, 1522. [CrossRef]
84. Liu, B.; Li, J.; Chen, B.; Shuai, Y.; He, X.; Liu, K.; He, M.; Jin, L. Dental pulp stem cells induce anti-inflammatory phenotypic transformation of macrophages to enhance osteogenic potential via IL-6/GP130/STAT3 signaling. *Ann. Transl. Med.* **2023**, *11*, 90. [CrossRef] [PubMed]
85. Jung, M.; Ma, Y.; Iyer, R.P.; DeLeon-Pennell, K.Y.; Yabluchanskiy, A.; Garrett, M.R.; Lindsey, M.L. IL-10 improves cardiac remodeling after myocardial infarction by stimulating M2 macrophage polarization and fibroblast activation. *Basic. Res. Cardiol.* **2017**, *112*, 33. [CrossRef] [PubMed]
86. Mahmoud, N.N.; Hamad, K.; Al Shibitini, A.; Juma, S.; Sharifi, S.; Gould, L.; Mahmoudi, M. Investigating Inflammatory Markers in Wound Healing: Understanding Implications and Identifying Artifacts. *ACS Pharmacol. Transl. Sci.* **2024**, *7*, 18–27. [CrossRef] [PubMed]
87. Zhang, C.; Han, Y.; Miao, L.; Yue, Z.; Xu, M.; Liu, K.; Hou, J. Human β-defensins are correlated with the immune infiltration and regulated by vitamin D(3) in periodontitis. *J. Periodontal Res.* **2023**, *58*, 986–996. [CrossRef] [PubMed]
88. Sadiqa, A.; Khan, M.K. Mediators of Periodontitis complementing the development of Neural Disorders. *Pak. J. Med. Sci.* **2024**, *40*, 214–221. [CrossRef]
89. Wadhwa, S.; Finn, T.R.; Kister, K.; Matsumura, S.; Levit, M.; Cantos, A.; Shah, J.; Bohn, B.; Lalla, E.; Grbic, J.T.; et al. Post-menopausal women with HIV have increased tooth loss. *BMC Oral. Health* **2024**, *24*, 52. [CrossRef]
90. Howell, M.D.; Boguniewicz, M.; Pastore, S.; Novak, N.; Bieber, T.; Girolomoni, G.; Leung, D.Y. Mechanism of HBD-3 deficiency in atopic dermatitis. *Clin. Immunol.* **2006**, *121*, 332–338. [CrossRef]
91. Ozola, L.; Pilmane, M. Local Defense Factors in Cleft-Affected Palate in Children before and during Milk Dentition Age: A Pilot Study. *J. Pers. Med.* **2023**, *14*, 27. [CrossRef]

Journal of
*Personalized
Medicine*

MDPI

Article

Long-Term Clinical Outcomes of 3D-Printed Subperiosteal Titanium Implants: A 6-Year Follow-Up

Neculai Onică [1,†], Dana Gabriela Budală [2,†], Elena-Raluca Baciu [2,*], Cezara Andreea Onică [1,*], Gabriela Luminița Gelețu [1], Alice Murariu [1], Mihail Balan [1], Mihaela Pertea [3] and Carmen Stelea [1]

1 Department of Surgery, Faculty of Dental Medicine, University of Medicine and Pharmacy "Grigore T. Popa", 700115 Iasi, Romania; onica_neculai@d.umfiasi.ro (N.O.); gabriela.geletu@umfiasi.ro (G.L.G.); alice.murariu@umfiasi.ro (A.M.); mihail.balan@umfiasi.ro (M.B.); carmen.stelea@umfiasi.ro (C.S.)

2 Department of Implantology, Removable Dentures, Dental Technology, Faculty of Dental Medicine, University of Medicine and Pharmacy "Grigore T. Popa", 700115 Iasi, Romania; dana-gabriela.bosinceanu@umfiasi.ro

3 Department of Plastic Surgery, Faculty of Medicine, University of Medicine and Pharmacy "Grigore T. Popa", 700115 Iasi, Romania; mihaela.pertea@umfiasi.ro

* Correspondence: elena.baciu@umfiasi.ro (E.-R.B.); cezara-andreea.onica@umfiasi.ro (C.A.O.)

† These authors contributed equally to this work.

Abstract: As an alternative to regenerative therapies, numerous authors have recently proposed bringing back subperiosteal implants. The aim of the study was to present our clinical experience with a subperiosteal jaw implant that needs minimal bone preparation and enables the rapid implantation of prosthetic teeth in edentulous, atrophic alveolar bone. The research included 36 complete or partial edentulous patients (61 subperiostal implants) over a period of 6 years. To create the patient-specific subperiostal implants design, DentalCAD 3.0 Galway software (exocad GmbH, Darmstadt, Germany) was used and fabricated with a Mysint 100 (Sisma S.p.A., Piovene Rocchette, Italy) by titanium alloy powder. The results showed that only 9 of the 36 cases were successful at 6-year follow-up, while 27 cases had complications, including exposure of the metal frame (early or delayed), mobility of the device prior to the first 4–6 months, and late mobility due to recurrent infections and progressive structure exposure; 1 case failed for reasons unrelated to the device. This study indicated that the prudent application of fully customized subperiosteal jaw implants is a dependable alternative for the dental rehabilitation of atrophic edentulous cases that necessitate bone grafts for traditional fixed dental implant solutions.

Keywords: subperiosteal implants; edentulous; complications

1. Introduction

Extremely edentulous maxilla and mandibular atrophy have made dental prosthesis rehabilitation very difficult [1]. Due to the high prevalence of compromised elderly patients with serious medical conditions, many patients with atrophic edentulous jaws, particularly the most severe Cawood and Howell Class VI cases [2], may never have access to a fixed dental prosthetic solution that would greatly enhance their quality of life. The long-term survival rate of endosseous implants is considered to be remarkable [3,4]. However, a certain quantity and quality of bone are needed for its installation [5]. Bone grafts, jaw osteotomies, sinus lifts, distractions of the alveolar ridge, zygomatic implants, and barrier membranes are traditionally used in complex reconstructive surgery for dental rehabilitation of atrophic edentulous jaws and alveoli, which is necessary for patients undergoing oncology or post-traumatic treatment [2,6,7]. The main drawbacks, without a doubt, are the long times between treatment initiation and final prosthesis delivery, the high morbidity rate, and the complex and time-consuming procedure [8–10].

Oral and maxillofacial surgery has made significant strides forward with the integration of computer-aided design (CAD) and computer-aided manufacturing (CAM) systems.

This technological leap has not only optimized the fabrication process but has also been a catalyst for innovation within the field. Among the numerous advances, the development of patient-specific implants (PSIs) stands out. These implants are tailored to the unique anatomical requirements of each patient, providing superior fit and function compared to traditional implants.

The advent of a new generation of subperiosteal patient-specific implants is one of the most noteworthy outcomes of this technological hype [11]. These implants offer a viable solution for patients with inadequate bone height who are not candidates for traditional endosseous implants without undergoing extensive bone grafting or augmentation procedures. However, the challenges related to inadequate mucoperiosteal integration are largely determined by the gingival biotype, which affects the quality and the volume, pertaining to the quantity of the overlying soft tissues [12]. Typically, significant bone resorption is accompanied by comparable reductions in soft tissue, supporting the notion that the soft tissue follows the bone. Additionally, given that subperiosteal implants are prescribed for cases with severe bone loss, the quality of the underlying bone is crucial for the long-term viability of the implants.

The surge in popularity of these subperiosteal PSIs can be attributed to their minimally invasive nature and the reduced surgical morbidity associated with their placement. The use of CAD/CAM technology in their design ensures highly accurate adaptation to the bone surface, which is critical for the stability and long-term success of the implant. Furthermore, this technology has facilitated the manufacturing of these complex structures with precision and efficiency, allowing for shorter production times and lower costs. Worldwide studies [13–18] have reported promising outcomes, with numerous patients experiencing enhancements in oral function, aesthetic satisfaction, and overall quality of life.

Implant failure can be attributed to suboptimal adaptation at the time of surgical placement, leading to potential implant mobilization or instability, structural fracture, infectious processes, or a diminution of osseous support in the absence of infection.

The objective of the research was to report the clinical findings obtained from a six-year follow-up of clinical cases, focusing on the complications of 3D-printed subperiosteal titanium implants used in the fixed prosthetic restoration of atrophic jaws.

2. Materials and Methods

2.1. Study Design and Patient Selection Criteria

During the interval from March 2017 to January 2018, 54 patients presented to the private Oral and Maxillofacial Surgery Centre with total and partial edentulism. However, 36 patients were eligible for treatment with custom fabricated DMLS (Direct Metal Laser Sintering) titanium subperiosteal implants.

Eligibility for participation was based on the following inclusion criteria:

- Age over 60 years, or younger individuals with severe bone loss, thin zygomas (<4 mm), or reduced vertical height, making it extremely challenging to place two zygomatic implants on the same side;
- Stable general and oral health status;
- Good oral hygiene;
- Complete or significantly partial edentulism accompanied by severe bone atrophy, which precludes the placement of standard-size implants;
- Opting out of bone regeneration procedures;
- Consent to attend postoperative follow-up appointments.

The exclusion criteria were as follows:

- Age under 60 years, except for the selected younger patients;
- Diagnosed with systemic diseases or receiving pharmacotherapy that contraindicates surgical intervention, including the following:
    - Immunocompromised state;
    - Uncontrolled diabetes mellitus;

    - Neoplasms of the head and neck region;
    - Undergoing bisphosphonate therapy;
    - Inadequate oral hygiene.
- Lifestyle habits such as tobacco use or bruxism;
- Less severe cases of partial or complete edentulism where the placement of standard-sized dental implants is feasible;
- Incapacity or unwillingness to adhere to requisite postoperative follow-up protocols.

The primary causes of tooth loss and jaw atrophy were severe periodontal disease and failure of conventional implants, which involved ongoing bone resorption around older implants.

All patients gave their informed consent after discussing the diagnosis, the outcomes with and without intervention, detailed therapeutic options, and the advantages, inherent risks, and possible complications associated with the treatment.

2.2. Pre-Surgical Cone-Beam Computed Tomography (CBCT)

Prior to clinical intervention, each participant underwent cone-beam computed tomography (CBCT) imaging. These CBCT scans were obtained utilizing Green X (Vatech, Hwaseong-si, Korea), operating under the parameters of a tube voltage of 60–99 kVp, tube current of 4–16 mA, and a focal spot size of 0.5 mm (Figure 1).

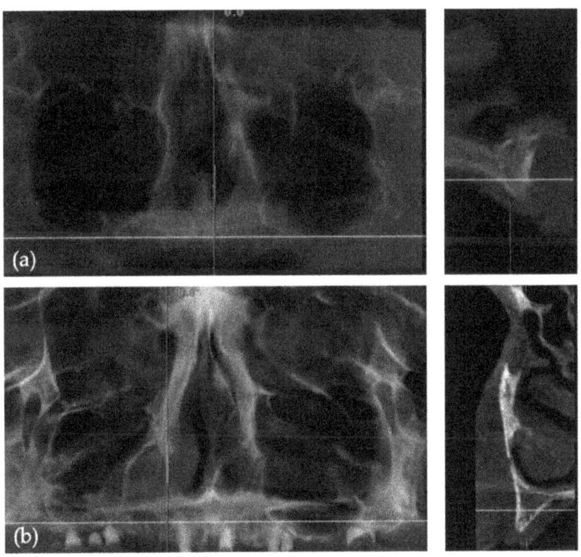

Figure 1. Pre-surgical CBCT images: (**a**,**b**) panoramic (green lines) and cross-sectional (red lines) views.

2.3. Design and Production of Patient-Specific Subperiostal Implants

Utilizing Exoplan 3.0 Galway software (Exocad GmbH, Darmstadt, Germany), the collected Digital Imaging and Communications in Medicine format (DICOM) data from the CBCT scans were processed to reconstruct the residual anatomical structure of the patient's bone in three dimensions; we subsequently saved the model as a standard tessellation (STL) file. Appropriate threshold values were meticulously selected to accurately render the cortical boundaries of the remaining bone. This process also included the strategic placement of the osseous fixation screws. Subsequently, the STL file underwent refinement within Exocad Galway 3.0 software (Exocad GmbH, Darmstadt, Germany), where descattering, removal of irregularities, and rectification of mesh anomalies were performed, thereby enhancing the visualization of the requisite prosthetic emergence profile and facilitating superior implant design.

Continuing within the same digital framework, the surgical cutting guide and the implant framework were constructed based on the STL files. Precise locations for the osteosynthesis screws were designated, and internal threading was incorporated to accommodate the multi-unit abutments. The edges were refined, surfaces were smoothed, angles were rounded, and the congruency of the implant with the bone surface was verified (Figure 2).

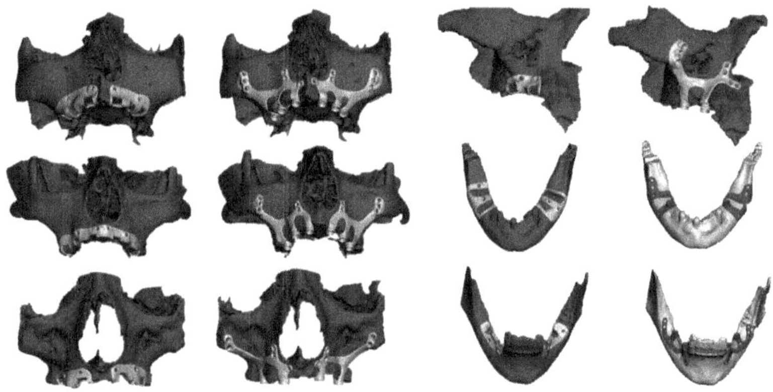

Figure 2. Three-dimensional virtual planning of different subperiosteal structures.

The comprehensive final designs were prepared for the manufacturing phase and subsequently sent to be printed with a DMLS system (Mysint 100, Sisma S.p.A., Piovene Rocchette, Italy) and titanium alloy powder (PowderRange Ti64, Carpenter Technology Corporation, Philadelphia, PA, USA). In total, 61 hybrid prostheses were fabricated (Table 1), and before packing and delivering, acid etching, plasma cleaning, and autoclave sterilization were performed.

Table 1. Characteristics of PSIs.

<table>
<tr><th>Location</th><th>Type</th><th>Number of Subperiosteal Structures</th><th>Number of Struts</th></tr>
<tr><td rowspan="3">Maxillary</td><td rowspan="2">Full arch</td><td>26</td><td>3 struts on a hemiarch</td></tr>
<tr><td>20</td><td>2 struts on a hemiarch</td></tr>
<tr><td>Partial
Uniterminal arch</td><td>2</td><td>2 struts</td></tr>
<tr><td rowspan="2">Mandibular</td><td>Partial
Biterminal arch</td><td>2 (×2)</td><td>2 struts on a hemiarch</td></tr>
<tr><td>Partial
Uniterminal arch</td><td>9</td><td>2 struts</td></tr>
</table>

2.4. Surgical Procedure and Prosthetic Treatment

The surgical procedures were typically conducted under local anesthesia (4% articaine with 1:100,000 epinephrine, Ubistein, 3M ESPE, St. Paul, MN, USA), with chairside monitoring and sedation administered by an anesthesiologist. The operative technique involved a crestal incision followed by adequate reflection of the periosteal flap, facilitating the placement of the implant. The bone-cutting guide was utilized for precise adaptation and positioning of the structure (Figure 3). Subsequent bone reduction and implant insertion were performed upon removal of the guide.

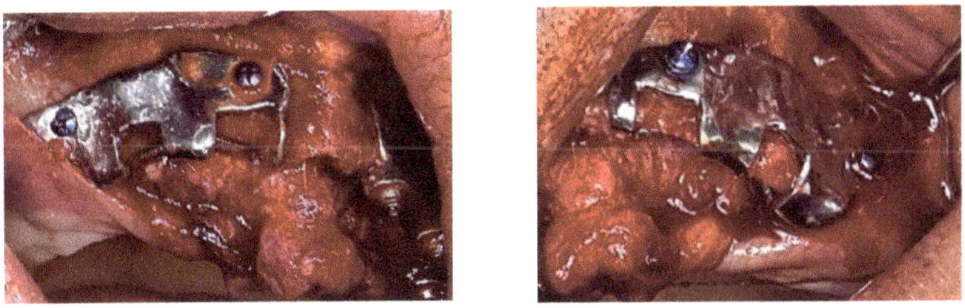

Figure 3. Intraoperative view of bone reduction guide.

When affixing the structure to the bone, self-drilling screws (Medicon eG, Tuttlingen, Germany) with a diameter of 2 mm were typically employed (Figure 4).

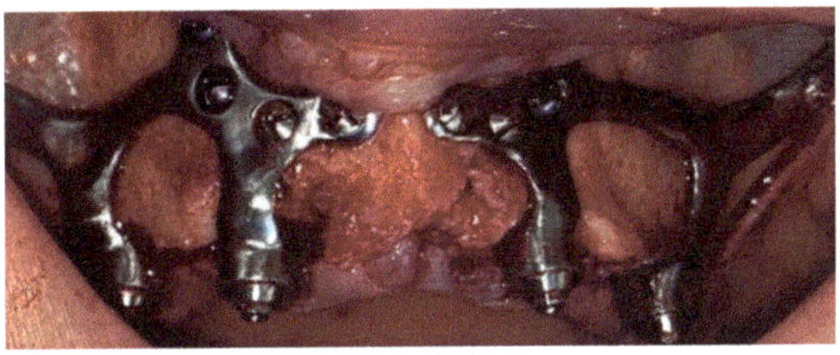

Figure 4. Intraoperative image showing two subperiosteal implants positioned and stabilized with screws.

The screws' lengths varied, extending from 5.5 to 9 mm in the paranasal and sub-spinal regions and from 11 mm to 13 mm within the zygomatic bone. Despite the self-drilling nature of the screws utilized in zygomatic applications, pre-drilling was executed to prepare the site. The protocol for screw insertion generally commenced with one screw at the anterior pillar, followed by the placement of 2 to 3 screws into the zygomatic bone, and concluding with the remaining screws in the paranasal and sub-spinal areas.

Occasionally, contingent upon clinical requirements, 1 to 2 palatal screws were positioned on each side. In the mandibular procedures, placement of screws on the lingual side was not practiced. Following the structural placement, a slow-resorbing membrane (Mucoderm) was applied to augment soft tissue thickness and prevent or delay potential exposure. The surgical site was closed with resorbable sutures.

For the first week after surgery, oral antibiotics (Augmentin, Glaxo Wellcome, Mayenne, France), analgesics, anti-inflammatories, and 0.12% chlorhexidine mouthwashes were administered two or three times a day.

The prosthetic rehabilitation involved taking impressions within 2 to 7 days after the surgical procedure for the provisional acrylic screw-retained prostheses. The impressions were obtained either traditional, using open-tray and polyether impression material (Impregum, 3 M ESPE, St. Paul, MN, USA) or digitally, with the CEREC Primescan intraoral optical scanner (Dentsply Sirona, Hanau, Germany). After 6 to 12 months following surgery, the final fixed restorations were performed using CAD/CAM milling technology.

Postoperative CBCT imaging was performed to ensure accurate positioning of the structure and to verify the precise placement of the screws.

2.5. Evaluating Complications and Implant Survival

In this study, the evaluated metrics encompassed immediate, early, and late postoperative complications. The last two types were further classified into minor and major complications. Minor complications included issues like exposure and infection. Major complications encompassed more severe problems such as recurrent infection, mobilization, and fracture of the structure, leading to the structure removal.

Immediate complications were defined as any immediate or secondary adverse event, such as discomfort, swelling, edema, or hemorrhage, that manifested within the initial two weeks after surgery, prior to the placement of the initial temporary restoration. These complications were of a biological origin.

Early complications refer to any issues that occurred during the period between the provisional and final restoration of a dental procedure. The three main complications may include infection, exposure, and mobilization. Common contributing factors to these problems often include improper fitting dental prostheses, an insufficient number of retention units, compromised bone density, and inadequate oral hygiene practices.

Late complications were any biological issues that developed following the delivery of the final prosthetic restoration until the 3-year follow-up. These issues could be of biological origin. Serious and/or recurring infections, with exudation or suppuration, discomfort, swelling, or pus development, with or without radiographic evidence of bone loss, are examples of late biological consequences. Late mobilization of the structure is due to the screw loosening after recurrent infections and insufficient mucoperiosteal and bony integration.

Subperiosteal implants deemed successful at the 6-year follow-up exhibited uninterrupted function without biological complications such as mucositis, exposure, or recurrent infection. Conversely, implants that required removal were categorized as failures. The survival rate included successful implants as well as those with manifestations of exposure and one to two infectious episodes, which remain under clinical monitoring.

2.6. Statistical Analysis

Statistical analysis was performed using IBM Statistical Package for the Social Sciences (SPSS) software (SPSS Inc., Chicago, IL, USA, version 26.0 for Windows). Descriptive data were analyzed using frequency and crosstabulation.

3. Results

The gender distribution in the study sample was 17 females (47.2%) and 19 males (52.8%). The ages ranged from 38 to 71 years, with a mean age of 61.9 ± 11.7 years. The characteristics of the study participants are presented in Table 2.

Table 2. Characteristics of initial study participants (N = 36).

Variables	Number	Percent [%]
Gender		
Male	19	52.8
Female	17	47.2
Age (mean ± SD [1])	61.9 ±11.7	
60 years and under	5	13.9
Over 60 years	31	86.1
Edentulism		
Completely or partially edentulous maxilla	25	16.7
Partially edentulous mandible	11	13.9
Patient-specific implant location		
Maxillary	48	78.7
Mandibular	13	21.3

[1] SD: standard deviation.

From the initial 36 patients, salvage of the PSIs was not an option in 15 cases due to severe infectious episodes, pain and discomfort, and progressive mobility (see Figure 5 and Table 3). Some of the cases with more stable results but with progressive exposure were addressed between 18 and 24 months with very poor outcomes. The surgical interventions only hastened the progression of the exposure, leading to further complications and making salvage surgery basically useless.

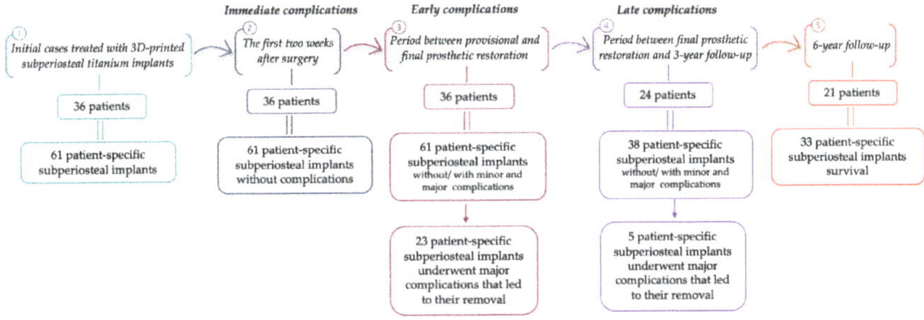

Figure 5. Schematic representation of the evolution of the cases included in the study.

Table 3. Characteristics of PSI complication.

Variables	Number	Percent [%]
Immediate complications		
Without complications	61	100
Implant survival	61	100
Early complications		
Without complications	20	32.8
Minor complications	18	29.5
Major complications with structure removal	23	37.7
Implant survival	38	62.3
Late complications		
Without complications	12	31.6
Minor complications	21	55.3
Major complications with structure removal	5	13.2
Implant survival	33	54.1
6-year follow-up		
Patient-specific implant success	12	36.4
Monitoring the patient-specific implant	21	63.6
Implant survival	33	54.1

After a 24-month period, progressive exposure was observed in eight patients in areas where adequate oral hygiene could not be maintained (Figure 6).

At the 6-year follow-up, structural removal was necessary for 15 patients. Currently, 12 patients remain under surveillance, while 9 patients have shown no complications. In the group under observation, we noted a soft tissue recession ranging from 2 to 4 mm, leading to slight exposure of the structural supports, predominantly on the buccal side (Figure 7).

The incidence of early complications (both minor and major) was 67.2% for a total of 61 PSIs, while the incidence of late complications was 68.4% for 38 PSIs. Statistical analysis revealed no significant differences in the occurrence of complications based on patient gender and age (Table 4). However, there were statistical differences in late complications and 6-year follow-up, associated with the implant location.

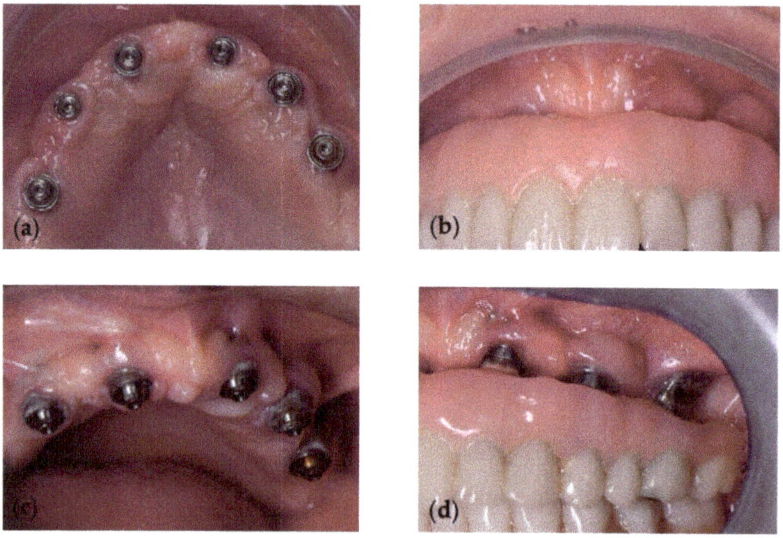

Figure 6. Intraoral aspect at (**a**,**b**) 24 months and (**c**,**d**) 42 months.

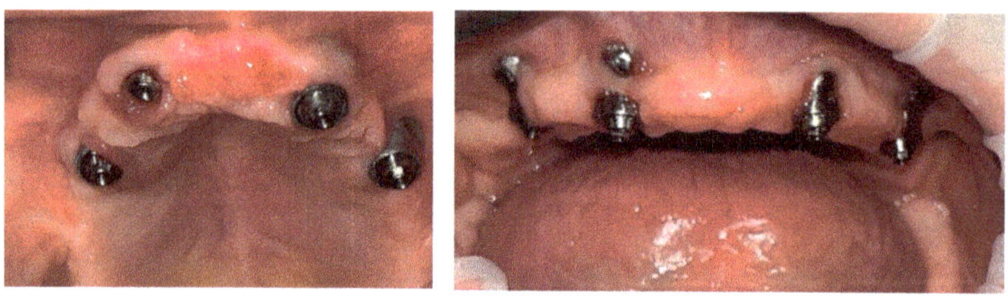

Figure 7. Intraoral examination at 6-year follow-up: minor complication involving soft tissue recession and exposure of structural supports.

Table 4. Aspects of the complication's appearance.

Variables		Early Complications (N, %)			Late Complications (N, %)			6-Year Follow-up (N, %)		
		Without	With	*p*-Value	Without	With	*p*-Value	Without	With	*p*-Value
Gender	Male	7 (36.8%)	12 (63.2%)	0.637	4 (30.8%)	9 (69.2%)	0.459	4 (36.4%)	7 (63.6%)	0.528
	Female	5 (29.4%)	12 (70.6%)		5 (45.5%)	6 (54.5%)		5 (50%)	5 (50%)	
	Total	12 (33.3%)	24 (66.7%)	-	9 (37.5%)	15 (62.5%)	-	9 (42.9%)	12 (57.1%)	
Age	≤60 years	2 (40%)	3 (60%)	0.733	1 (50%)	1 (50%)	0.803	1 (50%)	1 (50%)	0.830
	>60 years	10 (32.3%)	21 (67.7%)		9 (40.9%)	13 (59.1%)		8 (42.1%)	11 (57.9%)	
	Total	12 (33.3%)	24 (66.7%)	-	10 (41.7%)	14 (58.3%)		9 (42.9%)	12 (57.1%)	
Location	Maxillary	16 (33.3%)	32 (66.7%)	0.861	4 (15.4%)	22 (84.6%)	0.002 *	4 (18.2%)	18 (81.8%)	0.002 *
	Mandibular	4 (30.8%)	9 (69.2%)		8 (66.7%)	4 (33.3%)		8 (72.7%)	3 (27.3%)	
	Total	20 (32.8%)	41 (67.2%)	-	12 (31.6%)	26 (68.4%)		12 (36.4%)	21 (63.6%)	-

* Significance level of 0.05 (Chi-square test).

4. Discussion

The purpose of this publication was to convey our 6-year clinical observations with a novel, digitally custom-designed subperiosteal jaw implant. This technique was mainly addressed to patients with severe bone resorption in which bone grafting would be highly unpredictable due to the decreased osteogenic capacity of the recipient site, especially those with Cawood and Howell Class IV to VI edentulous ridges [2,7,18,19].

Historically, lost wax casting was the method of choice for manufacturing subperiosteal implants. However, issues with this process could compromise the clinical outcome and the final implant-to-bone fit [20]. In recent years, the adoption of CAD-CAM technologies and advanced manufacturing techniques like Direct Metal Laser Sintering (DMLS) and Selective Laser Melting (SLM) have facilitated the design and fabrication of these implants. These additive manufacturing processes allow for high precision in replicating the digitally generated STL file, significantly enhancing the fit and reducing human error [21–24]. Modern tools like DICOM cone-beam CT images and software such as Exoplan and Exocad 3.0 Galway have revolutionized the design process in virtual space, eliminating the need for physical alterations [25,26].

The clinical protocol has evolved from taking direct impressions of surgically exposed bone to installing heavy frames designed through digital workflows. This change has not only improved the healing process but has also enhanced the success rates of these devices [23,27]. The literature suggests that when standard implants are not suitable or extensive bone regeneration procedures are necessary, customized subperiosteal implants should be considered [27,28]. These implants are particularly beneficial as they can be loaded immediately, accelerating the recovery of function and quality of life for patients [29–31]. Typically, these implants support either fixed full-arch prostheses or partial-arch restorations and have successfully rehabilitated edentulous patients when used in retained overdentures [10].

Furthermore, multiple centers have documented innovative designs and applications of the new generation subperiosteal implant, showing the potential of multiple separate units to reconstruct a full arch, whereas a single unit may suffice for partial edentulous arches [13–17]. Our device is composed of 2 units to reconstruct a full arch and a single unit to reconstruct a partial edentulous arch. However, despite positive reviews, the literature lacks comprehensive data, with many studies reporting on a limited number of patients followed for insufficient periods [13,15]. The absence of multicenter clinical trials with long-term outcome data raises questions about the safety and efficacy of these implants on a broader scale.

A complete preoperative diagnosis remains crucial for a successful outcome. Prior to surgical treatment, thorough patient history collection, intraoral and extraoral examinations, high-quality CT scans, and meticulous prosthetic planning are essential to mitigate risks of biological and mechanical complications such as soft tissue dehiscence, peri-implantitis, or fractures. The integration of printed models and digital planning also plays a significant role in minimizing fitting issues, which are critical for the structural stability of the implants [28]. It is also essential to consider both surgical and prosthodontic factors meticulously, ensuring that the final prosthesis is designed with precision. Although some studies have suggested that cone-beam computed tomography provides adequate results [28], a high-quality CT scan is generally required for these fully customized implants to ensure they are perfectly tailored to the patient's anatomy [32].

Our study found a 62.3% survival rate for implants (including minor complications) in the first 3 years, with a 45.9% failure rate at the 6-year follow-up. This contrasts with findings from other studies. In a pilot study involving 16 patients, Nemtoi et al. [33] observed that after 6 months, only one custom-made DMLS subperiosteal maxillary implant failed, while 75% of the implants demonstrated a good to excellent fit. Mangano et al. [34] reported a perfect survival rate in their one-year study of ten patients, with a 10% incidence of early complications and a 20% incidence of late complications. Similarly, a prospective clinical investigation by Mounir et al. [35] reported a 100% survival rate after one year among ten patients, divided into two groups based on the material of the subperiosteal implants: Ti6Al4V alloy and Polyetheretherketone (PEEK), with five patients in each group. Furthermore, the retrospective analysis by Cerea et al. [21], which included the largest cohort of 70 patients and had the longest follow-up period of at least two years, showed a 95.8% implant survival rate with a 1.4% incidence of biological problems and an 8.9% incidence of mechanical issues.

Regarding gender, we found no difference in outcomes between male patients and females, even though all the females were postmenopausal (without bisphosphonate therapy). The explanation might be that, although females experience accelerated alveolar bone resorption and decreased bone mineral density due to osteoporosis, the impact may be offset by poorer hygiene practices and less frequent maintenance visits observed in male patients.

In younger individuals (under 60 years old), we observed inflammatory phenomena with an early onset and increased aggressiveness compared to others. This aspect can be attributed to an enhanced reactivity of the body to foreign bodies.

Based on our findings, early complications may arise from several directly involved factors, some of which are related to the structure of the implant, while others pertain to the patient. In terms of the structural integrity, there are two critical aspects that ensure the primary and long-term stability of the subperiosteal implant:

1. The precise fitting of the titanium frame to the bony surface (Figure 8). CAD-CAM technology typically provides accurate structures if the equipment, from CBCT to additive manufacturing, is calibrated correctly. Thus, the human factor remains the primary variable affecting the outcome.

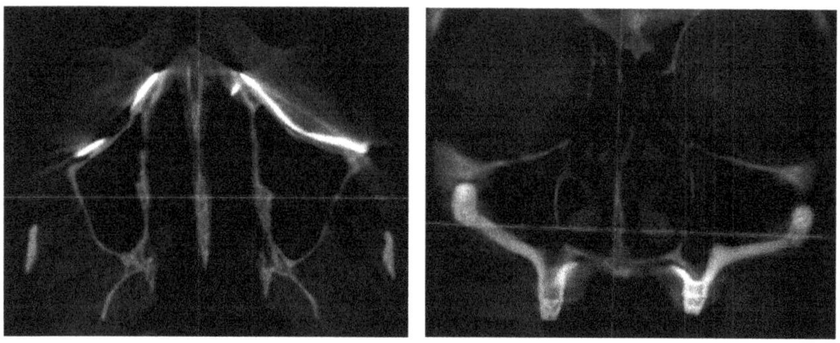

Figure 8. Radiographic images of a properly fitted dental implant at the two-year follow-up.

2. A sufficient number of screws should be placed in the most optimal positions within thick pillars and buttresses (Figure 9). The screws may be as long as the clinical situation permits, with a preference for bicortical placement. We recommend using at least four screws in the anterior pillar, with at least two positioned at the lower pole of the piriform rim, measuring 2/9 mm. Additionally, at least two screws should be anchored in the zygomatic bone, with a minimum size of 2/11 mm. Stefano et al. [36] suggested in their case report that for the canine fossa and zygomatic bone, screws measuring 6 to 8 mm are necessary to allow for stable fixation. Self-drilling screws appear to provide better primary stability than self-tapping screws. Regardless of the screw type, predrilling at the zygomatic bone anchorage is essential.

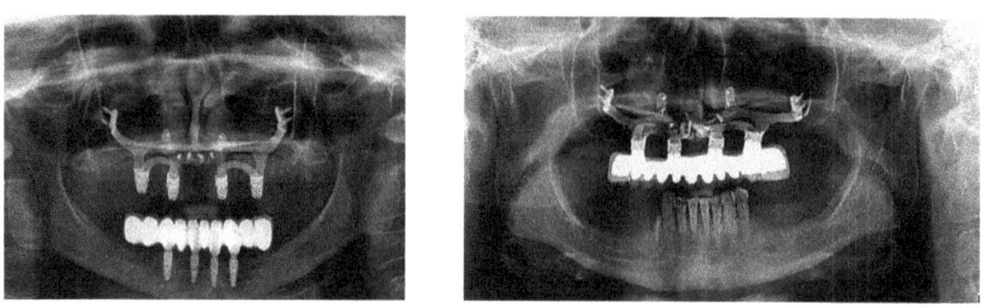

Figure 9. A sufficient number of screws can prevent future mobilization of the structure.

3. The number of struts can significantly impact long-term soft tissue stability. Faster and more pronounced exposure has been observed in structures with three struts on a hemiarch compared to those with two struts.

The present study is limited by the small number of patients included and the absence of consensus on the design of PSIs, their indications based on bone quality, and the optimal positioning and number of screws required to achieve both primary and long-term stability. Despite promising advancements in subperiosteal implant technology have shown promising results, the limited clinical data available highlight the need for further research. Future studies should focus on increasing the sample size and extending follow-up periods to fully assess the viability of these advanced implant solutions.

5. Conclusions

Our results, showing a 25% (9 patients from 36 initial) success rate at the 6-year follow-up, indicate that subperiosteal implant-supported hybrid prostheses, designed via digital planning and guided surgery, have proven unsatisfactory and remain a questionable option for long-term treatment. There is a need for additional research into the biocompatibility of the materials used, the design of the structure, and how the body reacts to it.

Author Contributions: Conceptualization, N.O. and D.G.B.; methodology N.O. and D.G.B.; validation, A.M.; investigation, N.O. and D.G.B.; resources, G.L.G. and M.B.; writing—original draft preparation, N.O., D.G.B. and E.-R.B.; writing—review and editing, E.-R.B. and C.A.O.; visualization, M.P.; supervision, N.O. and D.G.B.; project administration, C.S. All authors have read and agreed to the published version of the manuscript.

Funding: This research received no external funding.

Institutional Review Board Statement: This study did not require ethical approval. The surgical procedures were performed in accordance with the protocols, guidelines, and ethical practices established by the medical community to ensure patient safety, optimal outcomes, and ethical treatment.

Informed Consent Statement: Informed consents were obtained from the subjects involved in this study. Written informed consent was obtained from the patients prior to the publication of this paper.

Data Availability Statement: The original contributions presented in the study are included in the article, further inquiries can be directed to the corresponding authors.

Conflicts of Interest: The authors declare no conflicts of interest.

References

1. Kern, J.S.; Kern, T.; Wolfart, S.; Heussen, N. A systematic review and meta-analysis of removable and fixed implant-supported prostheses in edentulous jaws: Post-loading implant loss. *Clin. Oral Implants Res.* **2016**, *27*, 174–195. [CrossRef] [PubMed]
2. Cawood, J.I.; Howell, R.A. A classification of the edentulous jaws. *Int. J. Oral Maxillofac. Surg.* **1988**, *17*, 232–236. [CrossRef] [PubMed]
3. Buser, D.; Sennerby, L.; De Bruyn, H. Modern implant dentistry based on osseointegration: 50 years of progress, current trends and open questions. *Periodontol. 2000* **2017**, *73*, 7–21. [CrossRef] [PubMed]
4. Chatzopoulos, G.S.; Wolff, L.F. Retrospective analysis of 50,333 implants on implant failure and associated patient-related factors. *J. Stomatol. Oral Maxillofac. Surg.* **2023**, *124* (Suppl. S6), 101555. [CrossRef] [PubMed]
5. Zheng, Z.; Ao, X.; Xie, P.; Jiang, F.; Chen, W. The biological width around implant. *J. Prosthodont. Res.* **2021**, *65*, 11–18. [CrossRef] [PubMed]
6. Keleş, H.G.; Karaca, Ç. Comparison of Stress Distribution Among Standard Dental Implants Placed in Grafted Bone, Zygomatic Implants, and Subperiosteal Implants in the Atrophic Edentulous Maxilla: 3D Finite Element Analysis. *Int. J. Oral Maxillofac. Implants* **2023**, *38*, 347–356. [CrossRef]
7. Anitua, E.; Eguia, A.; Staudigl, C.; Alkhraisat, M.H. Clinical performance of additively manufactured subperiosteal implants: A systematic review. *Int. J. Implant. Dent.* **2024**, *10*, 4. [CrossRef]
8. Herce-López, J.; Pingarrón, M.D.C.; Tofé-Povedano, Á.; García-Arana, L.; Espino-Segura-Illa, M.; Sieira-Gil, R.; Rodado-Alonso, C.; Sánchez-Torres, A.; Figueiredo, R. Customized Subperiosteal Implants for the Rehabilitation of Atrophic Jaws: A Consensus Report and Literature Review. *Biomimetics* **2024**, *9*, 61. [CrossRef] [PubMed]

9. Tofé-Povedano, A.; Parras-Hernández, J.; Herce-López, J.; Matute-García, D.; González-Moguena, V.A.; Rollón-Mayordomo, A. Design modifications in subperiosteal implants to avoid complications. Presentation of a case series study and literature review. *Rev. Esp. Cir. Oral Maxilofac.* **2023**, *45*, 57–63.
10. Vatteroni, E.; Covani, U.; Menchini Fabris, G.B. The New Generation of Subperiosteal Implants for Patient-Specific Treatment of Atrophic Dental Arches: Literature Review and Two Case Reports. *Int. J. Periodontics Restor. Dent.* **2023**, *43*, 735–741. [CrossRef]
11. Dimitroulis, G.; Gupta, B.; Wilson, I.; Hart, C. The atrophic edentulous alveolus. A preliminary study on a new generation of subperiosteal implants. *Oral Maxillofac. Surg.* **2023**, *27*, 69–78. [CrossRef] [PubMed]
12. Van den Borre, C.; De Neef, B.; Loomans, N.A.J.; Rinaldi, M.; Nout, E.; Bouvry, P.; Naert, I.; Van Stralen, K.J.; Mommaerts, M.Y. Soft Tissue Response and Determination of Underlying Risk Drivers for Recession and Mucositis after AMSJI Implantation in the Maxilla. *Int. J. Oral Maxillofac. Implants* **2024**, *39*, 302–309. [CrossRef] [PubMed]
13. Chochlidakis, K.; Einarsdottir, E.; Tsigarida, A.; Papaspyridakos, P.; Romeo, D.; Barmak, A.B.; Ercoli, C. Survival rates and prosthetic complications of implant fixed complete dental prostheses: An up to 5-year retrospective study. *J. Prosthet. Dent.* **2020**, *124*, 539–546. [CrossRef] [PubMed]
14. Minichetti, J.C. Analysis of HA-coated subperiosteal implants. *J. Oral Implantol.* **2003**, *29*, 111–116, discussion 117–119. [CrossRef] [PubMed]
15. Rutkowski, J.L.; Iyer, S. Occlusion and Dental Implants-Where Are We? *J. Oral Implantol.* **2023**, *49*, 229–232. [CrossRef]
16. Brånemark, P.I.; Hansson, B.O.; Adell, R.; Breine, U.; Lindström, J.; Hallén, O.; Ohman, A. Osseointegrated implants in the treatment of the edentulous jaw. Experience from a 10-year period. *Scand. J. Plast. Reconstr. Surg. Suppl.* **1977**, *16*, 1–132.
17. Spitznagel, F.A.; Balmer, M.; Wiedemeier, D.B.; Jung, R.E.; Gierthmuehlen, P.C. Clinical outcomes of all-ceramic single crowns and fixed dental prostheses supported by ceramic implants: A systematic review and meta-analyses. *Clin. Oral Implants Res.* **2022**, *33*, 1–20. [CrossRef] [PubMed]
18. Tolstunov, L.; Hamrick, J.F.E.; Broumand, V.; Shilo, D.; Rachmiel, A. Bone Augmentation Techniques for Horizontal and Vertical Alveolar Ridge Deficiency in Oral Implantology. *Oral Maxillofac. Surg. Clin. N. Am.* **2019**, *31*, 163–191. [CrossRef]
19. Sáez-Alcaide, L.M.; González Gallego, B.; Fernando Moreno, J.; Moreno Navarro, M.; Cobo-Vázquez, C.; Cortés-Bretón Brinkmann, J.; Meniz-García, C. Complications associated with vertical bone augmentation techniques in implant dentistry: A systematic review of clinical studies published in the last ten years. *J. Stomatol. Oral Maxillofac. Surg.* **2023**, *124*, 101574. [CrossRef]
20. Romanos, G.; Lau, J.; Zhang, Y.; Hou, W.; Delgado-Ruiz, R. Macrogeometry and Bone Density Control Over the Primary Stability of 6-mm Implants: An In Vitro Study. *Int. J. Oral Maxillofac. Implants* **2021**, *36*, 322–326. [CrossRef]
21. Cerea, M.; Dolcini, G.A. Custom-Made Direct Metal Laser Sintering Titanium Subperiosteal Implants: A Retrospective Clinical Study on 70 Patients. *BioMed Res. Int.* **2018**, *2018*, 5420391. [CrossRef] [PubMed]
22. Strappa, E.M.; Memè, L.; Cerea, M.; Roy, M.; Bambini, F. Custom-made additively manufactured subperiosteal implant. *Minerva Dent. Oral Sci.* **2022**, *71*, 353–360. [CrossRef] [PubMed]
23. Roy, M.; Corti, A.; Dominici, S.; Pompella, A.; Cerea, M.; Chelucci, E.; Dorocka-Bobkowska, B.; Daniele, S. Biocompatibility of Subperiosteal Dental Implants: Effects of Differently Treated Titanium Surfaces on the Expression of ECM-Related Genes in Gingival Fibroblasts. *J. Funct. Biomater.* **2023**, *14*, 59. [CrossRef] [PubMed]
24. Cohen, D.J.; Cheng, A.; Kahn, A.; Aviram, M.; Whitehead, A.J.; Hyzy, S.L.; Clohessy, R.M.; Boyan, B.D.; Schwartz, Z. Novel Osteogenic Ti-6Al-4V Device for Restoration of Dental Function In Patients With Large Bone Deficiencies: Design, Development And Implementation. *Sci. Rep.* **2016**, *6*, 20493. [CrossRef] [PubMed]
25. Block, M.S. Dental Implants: The Last 100 Years. *J. Oral Maxillofac. Surg.* **2018**, *76*, 11–26. [CrossRef] [PubMed]
26. Dal Carlo, L.; Pasqualini, M.; Shulman, M.; Rossi, F.; Comola, G.; Manenti, P.; Candotto, V.; Lauritano, D.; Zampetti, P. Endosseous distal extension (EDE) blade implant technique useful to provide stable pillars in the ipotrophic lower posterior sector: 22 years statistical survey. *Int. J. Immunopathol. Pharmacol.* **2019**, *33*, 2058738419838092. [CrossRef] [PubMed]
27. Mommaerts, M.Y. Evolutionary steps in the design and biofunctionalization of the additively manufactured sub-periosteal jaw implant 'AMSJI' for the maxilla. *Int. J. Oral Maxillofac. Implants* **2019**, *48*, 108–114. [CrossRef]
28. Carretero, J.L.C.; Vera, J.L.D.C.P.d.; García, N.M.; Martínez, P.G.; Martínez, M.M.P.; Niño, I.A.; Cuéllar, I.N.; Cuéllar, C.N. Virtual surgical planning and customized subperiosteal titanium maxillary implant (CSTMI) for three dimensional reconstruction and dental implants of maxillary defects after oncological resection: Case series. *J. Clin. Med.* **2022**, *11*, 4594. [CrossRef] [PubMed]
29. De Tapia, B.; Mozas, C.; Valles, C.; Nart, J.; Sanz, M.; Herrera, D. Adjunctive effect of modifying the implant-supported prosthesis in the treatment of peri-implant mucositis. *J. Clin. Periodontol.* **2019**, *46*, 1050–1060. [CrossRef]
30. Peev, S.; Sabeva, E. Subperiosteal implants in treatment of total and partial edentulism-A long term follow up. *Int. J. Sci. Res.* **2016**, *5*, 98–99.
31. Gellrich, N.C.; Rahlf, B.; Zimmerer, R.; Pott, P.C.; Rana, M. A new concept for implant-borne dental rehabilitation; how to overcome the biological weak-spot of conventional dental implants? *Head Face Med.* **2017**, *13*, 17. [CrossRef] [PubMed]
32. Surovas, A. A digital workflow for modeling of custom dental implants. *3D Print Med.* **2019**, *5*, 9. [CrossRef] [PubMed]
33. Nemtoi, A.; Covrig, V.; Nemtoi, A.; Stoica, G.; Vatavu, R.; Haba, D.; Zetu, I. Custom-Made Direct Metal Laser Sintering Titanium Subperiosteal Implants in Oral and Maxillofacial Surgery for Severe Bone-Deficient Patients-A Pilot Study. *Diagnostics* **2022**, *12*, 2531. [CrossRef] [PubMed]

34. Mangano, C.; Bianchi, A.; Mangano, F.G.; Dana, J.; Colombo, M.; Solop, I.; Admakin, O. Custom-made 3D printed subperiosteal titanium implants for the prosthetic restoration of the atrophic posterior mandible of elderly patients: A case series. *3D Print Med.* **2020**, *6*, 1. [CrossRef] [PubMed]
35. Mounir, M.; Atef, M.; Abou-Elfetouh, A.; Hakam, M.M. Titanium and polyether ether ketone (PEEK) patient-specific subperiosteal implants: Two novel approaches for rehabilitation of the severely atrophic anterior maxillary ridge. *Int. J. Oral Maxillofac. Surg.* **2018**, *47*, 658–664. [CrossRef]
36. Stefano, N.; Lorenzo, V. The Use of Digital Sub-Periosteal Implants in Severe Maxillary Atrophies Rehabilitation: A Case Report. *J. Head Neck Spine Surg.* **2021**, *4*, 555636.

Journal of *Personalized Medicine*

MDPI

Article

Comparison of Nasal Dimensions According to the Facial and Nasal Indices Using Cone-Beam Computed Tomography

Jeong-Hyun Lee [1,†], Hey-Suk Kim [2,†] and Jong-Tae Park [1,3,*]

1 Department of Oral Anatomy, Dankook Institute for Future Science and Emerging Convergence, Dental College, Dan-Kook University, Cheonan 31116, Republic of Korea; 911105jh@dankook.ac.kr
2 Department of Crime Scene Investigation Unit, Forensic Science Division, Daejeon Metropolitan Police, Daejeon 35403, Republic of Korea; kallaa@daum.net
3 Department of Bio Health Convergency Open Sharing System, Dan-Kook University, Cheonan 31116, Republic of Korea
* Correspondence: jongta2@dankook.ac.kr; Tel.: +82-41-550-1926
† These authors contributed equally to this work.

Abstract: The nasal cavity constitutes the foremost portion of the respiratory system, composed of the anterior nasal aperture, nostrils, and choanae. It has an intricate anatomical structure since it has various functions, such as heat exchange, humidification, and filtration. Accordingly, clinical symptoms related to the nose, such as nasal congestion, snoring, and nasal septal deviation, are closely linked to the complex anatomical structure of the nasal cavity. Thus, the nasal cavity stands as a paramount structure in both forensic and clinical contexts. The majority of relevant studies have performed comparisons between sexes, with studies making comparisons according to the FI and NI only and examining relative percentages. Furthermore, the nasal cavity was measured in 2D, and not 3D, in most cases. In this study, we conducted a 3D modeling and anthropometric assessment of the nasal cavity using a 3D analysis software. Furthermore, we aimed to investigate whether the size of the nasal cavity differs according to sex, facial index (FI), and nasal index (NI). We retrospectively reviewed the cone-beam computed tomography (CBCT) data of 100 participants (50 males, 50 females) aged 20–29 years who visited the dental hospital of Dankook University (IRB approval no. DKUDH IRB 2020-01-007). Our findings showed that nasal cavity sizes generally differed according to sex, FI, and NI. These findings provide implications for performing patient-tailored surgeries in clinical practice and conducting further research on the nasal cavity. Therefore, we believe that our study makes a significant contribution to the literature.

Keywords: nasal cavity; nasal index; facial index; CBCT; 3D modeling

1. Introduction

The nasal cavity constitutes the foremost portion of the respiratory system, composed of the anterior nasal aperture, nostrils, and choanae [1]. It has an intricate anatomical structure since it has various functions, such as heat exchange, humidification, and filtration [2]. Accordingly, clinical symptoms related to the nose, such as nasal congestion, snoring, and nasal septal deviation, are closely linked to the complex anatomical structure of the nasal cavity [2]. Forensic science has recently been trending towards determining the sex of unidentified skeletal remains and performing facial reconstruction [3–8]. Sex determination, in particular, primarily relies on anatomical features, including the pelvis, mastoid processes, and nasal cavity size [9–11]. Among these structures, the nasal cavity has been reported to be a useful auxiliary tool for personal identification and age estimation [12–14]. Thus, the nasal cavity stands as a paramount structure in both forensic and clinical contexts.

Cone-beam computed tomography (CBCT) technology is being used in many studies. Particularly, it allows for the observation of the complex craniofacial structure in 3D, enabling more precise analysis and diagnosis than traditional 2D methods [15]. As such, it is currently playing a central role in clinical research. Moreover, CBCT is now being utilized in the field of forensic science, unlike before. According to the research by Jayakrishnan [15], CBCT plays an important role in personal identification and facial reconstruction. Additionally, the study by Akbar et al. [16] conducted research on age estimation by measuring the dimensions and volume ratio of teeth using CBCT, and the studies by Azmi et al. [17] and Denny et al. [18] conducted gender analysis through the evaluation of the frontal sinus using CBCT. Thus, CBCT is being used as a tool necessary for identity verification in forensics, including age and gender. In light of this, this study also aims to conduct a analysis by modeling the nasal cavity in 3D, which is difficult to evaluate in 2D.

In contemporary society, facial contours have captured interest in foundational fields, such as anatomy and anthropology, as well as in clinical disciplines, such as plastic surgery. In forensic science, facial contours are essential structures for personal identification and sex determination [19]. Currently, there is ongoing research on the classifications of the facial index (FI) and nasal index (NI) [1–14,19–22]. FI classification differentiates facial shapes into hypereuryprosopic, euryprosopic, mesoprosopic, leptoprosopic, and hyperleptoprosopic based on facial length [20,21]. NI classification categorizes nose shapes into leptorrhine (long and narrow nose), mesorrhine (medium nose), and platyrrhine (broad nose) based on nasal length [22,23]. These facial and nasal shape classifications are being utilized not only in osteological assessments but also clinically [24–26].

Current research on the nasal cavity surpasses its forensic and clinical significance, also contributing to technological advancements in physical anthropology. The precision of measurements plays a critical role in advancing personal identification methodologies and enhancing our comprehension of human evolutionary processes. Consequently, this underscores the imperative need for research in three-dimensional technologies. Moreover, nasal cavity studies through 3D analysis enable a profound comprehension of nasal anatomy, offering the potential to significantly elevate the precision of clinical surgeries by addressing patient-specific anatomical discrepancies. This underscores the increasing importance of utilizing 3D technology in nasal research, necessitating further exploration in this field.

The majority of relevant studies have performed comparisons between sexes [1–14,19–38], with studies making comparisons according to the FI and NI only and examining relative percentages [1–14,19–22]. Furthermore, the nasal cavity was measured in 2D, and not 3D, in most cases [1–14,19–38]. However, the nasal cavity should be measured in 3D, as it consists of a roof, floor, medial wall, and lateral wall [1].

Mimics software is a program developed by Materialise, which is extensively utilized as an advanced medical imaging and 3D modeling tool in the medical industry. It easily converts medical scan data from CT and MRI scans into precise 3D models, enabling medical professionals to conduct more accurate diagnoses and create customized medical solutions for patients. The key utility of Mimics software lies in its ability to replicate accurate anatomical structures for patients, which is critically used for surgical planning, medical research, and educational purposes. For instance, surgeons utilize the 3D models provided by Mimics software to perform pre-surgical simulations, thereby preventing potential surgical risks and complications during actual operations. Furthermore, the software facilitates the development of customized medical devices and implants tailored to the unique anatomical structures of individual patients.

Mimics software provides a comprehensive suite of tools for the detailed analysis and measurement of anatomical structures. Users can utilize its advanced analytical tools to extract quantitative data, perform virtual surgeries, and evaluate procedural outcomes, offering a valuable resource for surgical planning and biomechanics research where understanding the interactions between different tissues and materials is essential.

Additionally, the software simplifies the complex process of 3D medical modeling, offering a user-friendly interface that makes it accessible for educational use. This ease of use allows students to employ the program effortlessly, enhancing their understanding of human biology and anatomical variations through hands-on experience with anatomical models.

In forensic medicine, Mimics is employed for personal identification purposes. It possesses applications for reconstructing unidentified remains, aiding forensic experts by modeling soft tissues over skeletal remains to deduce physical characteristics and potentially identify the deceased.

Overall, Mimics software provides essential tools for modern medical practices, including detailed anatomical visualization, custom implant design, surgical simulation, and educational applications. It represents a significant technological advancement in the medical field. To measure the complex structure of the nasal cavity, Mimics software was utilized.

In this context, this study aims to conduct a 3D modeling and anthropometric assessment of the nasal cavity using a 3D analysis software (Mimics, version 22.0, Materialise, Leuven, Belgium). Furthermore, we aim to investigate whether the size of the nasal cavity differs according to sex, FI, and NI. This study aims to provide data necessary not only for future medical approaches but also for significant implications from an anthropological perspective.

2. Materials and Methods

2.1. Study Population

The cone-beam computed tomography (CBCT) data of 100 participants (50 males, 50 females) aged 20–29 years who visited the dental hospital of Dankook University and had no tooth loss, asymmetry, or systemic diseases were obtained. The sample size was determined using the G-Power 3.1 (HHU, England) software. The data of patients whose treatments had already been completed were obtained for retrospective review; thus, an exemption from informed consent of this study was granted by the Institutional Review Board at Dankook University (IRB approval no. DKUDH IRB 2020-01-007).

2.2. Method

2.2.1. CBCT Data

The CBCT images were taken by one technician. The participants were scanned in a manner to ensure the perpendicular alignment of the Frankfort horizontal plane to the ground to minimize distortions of the nasal cavity size across the participants. In addition, the CT scanner (Alphard 3030, Asahi, Kyoto, Japan) was positioned to match the midline of the face, and imaging was performed using specific settings: gantry angle at 0°, voltage set at 120 kV, and auto mA conditions. The following parameters were used for the CBCT: a slice increment of 0.39 mm, a slice thickness of 0.39 mm, a slice pitch set to 3, a scanning time of 4 s, and a matrix of 512 px × 512 px for image resolution. The resulting CBCT data were received in DICOM format.

2.2.2. Mimics 3D Modeling

The CBCT DICOM files were processed using Mimics (version 22.0, Materialise, Leuven, Belgium) to extract 3D patient data. The 3D modeling was performed in three views (coronal view, sagittal view, and frontal view) for better precision. The Hounsfield Unit (HU) [23] value was adjusted for the 3D modeling.

(1) Cranial 3D modeling

The HU values for the skull were set within the designated average range in Mimics software (Mimics, version 22.0, Materialise, Leuven, Belgium), Min 500 HU and Max 3071 HU, for the masking process. Additionally, unnecessary noise, soft tissues, and bones were removed using the 'Edit mask' function. After removal, the completed data were converted to STL files using the 'CalCulate Part' function. Subsequently, for precise measurements, 'points' were created in the 'Analyze' section for each measurement item, and measurements were conducted for each item using the 'Distance' function.

(2) Nasal cavity 3D modeling

Since there is no predefined average range for the HU values of the nasal cavity in Mimics software, masking was conducted in custom mode. Initially, a new mask was created with settings at Min −1024 HU and Max −265 HU, and then to exclusively extract the nasal cavity, the 'Crop Mask' feature was used to set the region containing the nasal cavity in three views: coronal, sagittal, and frontal. Subsequently, the 'Edit mask' feature was used to remove noise. The completed data were converted to STL files using the 'CalCulate Part' function. For precise measurements, 'points' were created in the 'Analyze' section for each measurement item, and measurements were conducted for each item using the 'Distance' function.

(3) Soft tissue 3D modeling

The HU values for soft tissues were set within the designated average range in Mimics software, Min −390 HU and Max 160 HU, for the masking process. Additionally, unnecessary noise and bones were removed using the 'Edit mask' function. After removal, the completed data were converted to STL files using the 'CalCulate Part' function. For precise measurements, 'points' were created in the 'Analyze' section for each measurement item, and measurements were conducted for each item using the 'Distance' function.

2.2.3. Measurement Parameters

All measurements were taken after calibrating the Frankfort horizontal line for precision. To ensure accuracy, the analyze point feature was used to mark points and measure the distance between the points. The measurements were taken at the highest point. Two measurements were taken by Kim and Lee (one each), and the average values were calculated for a reliability assessment (Cronbach's $\alpha = 0.623$) before statistical analysis. Furthermore, FI and NI were computed based on the measurements.

(1) Facial index (FI)

The FI classifies facial appearance into five types based on facial height (FH) and facial width (FW). FH is the distance between the nasion (n) and gnathion (gn), and FW is the bizygomatic width (zygion–zygion) (Figure 1). Classifications were made using the formula: FH/FW × 100 [28]. Table 1 shows the classification results.

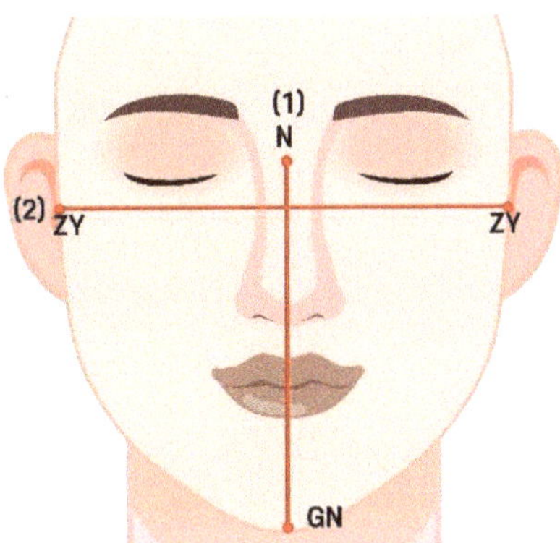

Figure 1. Facial index measurement. (1) FH is the distance between the nasion (n) and gnathion (gn); (2) FW is the bizygomatic width (zygion–zygion).

Table 1. Facial index classification.

Facial Index	Range of FI	N
Hypereuryprosopic (very broad face)	80%	75
Euryprosopic (broad face)	80~85%	20
Mesoprosopic (round face)	85~90%	5

(2) NI

The NI classifies the nasal appearance into five types based on the nasal width (NW) and nasal height (NH). NW is the distance between the alaria (al), and NH is the distance between the nasion (n) and subnasale (sn) (Figure 2). Classifications were made using the formula: NW/NH × 100 [29]. Table 2 shows the classification results.

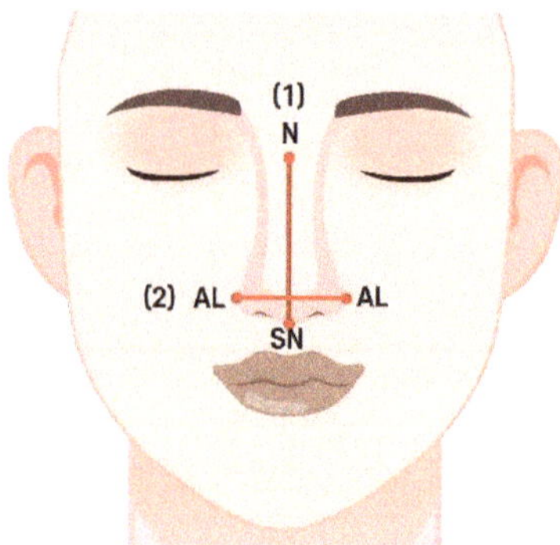

Figure 2. Facial index measurement. (1) NH is the distance between the nasion (n) and subnasale (sn); (2) NW is the distance between the alaria (al).

Table 2. Nasal index classification.

Nasal Index	Range of FI	N
Leptorrhine (long and narrow)	55~69.9%	10
Mesorrhine (moderate shape)	70~84.9%	76
Platyrrhine (broad and short)	85~99.9%	14

(3) Measurement parameters

The parameters that were measured for the nasal cavity are shown in Table 3 (Figures 3 and 4).

Table 3. Nasal cavity measurement parameters.

Parameter	Definition
Septum length	Width of the nasal septum in sagittal view
Septum height	Height of nasal septum in coronal view
Nasal cavity width	Width of nasal cavities in coronal view
Nasal cavity height	Height of nasal cavities in coronal view
Nasal cavity length	Width of nasal cavities in sagittal view

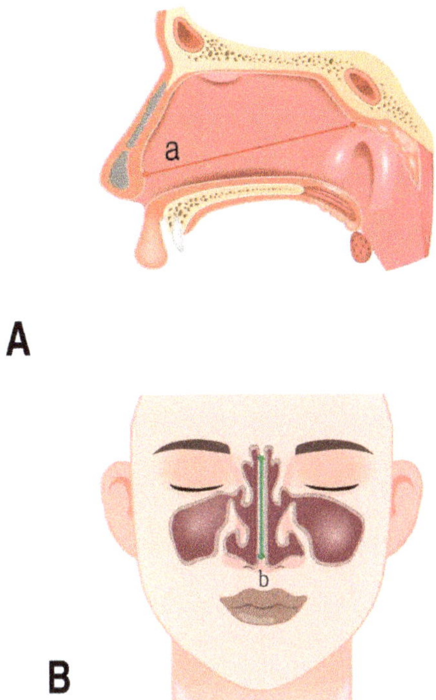

Figure 3. Septum measurement. (**A**) Septum length; a: the distance length of the highest point septum; (**B**) septum height; b: the distance height of the highest point septum.

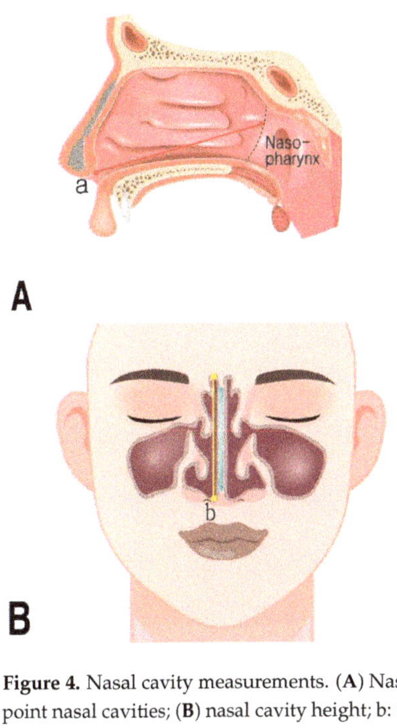

Figure 4. Nasal cavity measurements. (**A**) Nasal cavity length; a: the distance height of the highest point nasal cavities; (**B**) nasal cavity height; b: the distance length of the highest point nasal cavities.

2.2.4. Three-Dimensional Model Measurement in Mimics Software

The method of measuring patient CBCT data after 3D modeling is illustrated in Figures 5 and 6.

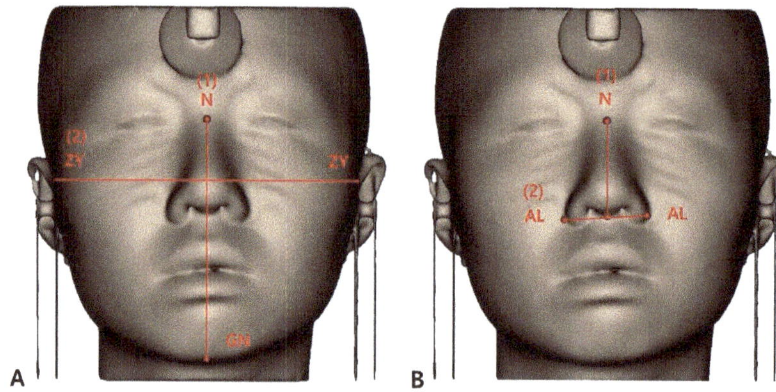

Figure 5. (**A**) Facial index measurement. (1) FH is the distance between the nasion (n) and gnathion (gn); (2) FW is the bizygomatic width (zygion–zygion). (**B**) Facial index measurement. (1) NH is the distance between the nasion (n) and subnasale (sn); (2) NW is the distance between the alaria (al).

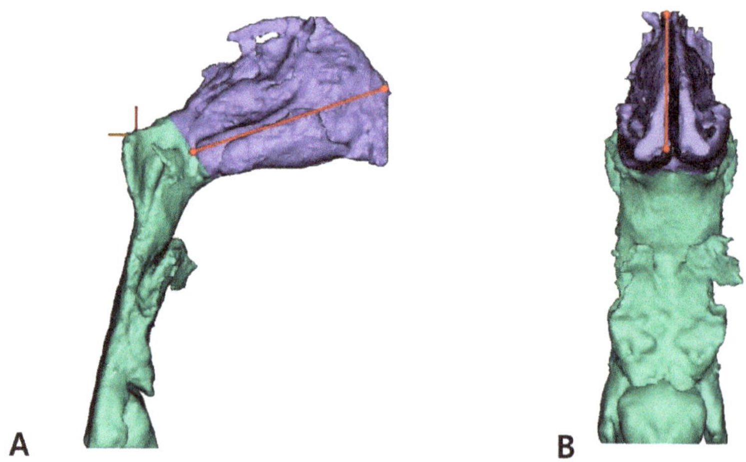

Figure 6. Nasal cavity measurements. (**A**) Nasal cavity length. (**B**) Nasal cavity height.

2.2.5. Statistics

Data were analyzed using IBM SPSS Statistics for Windows, version 23 (IBM Corp., Armonk, NY, USA). Differences in nasal cavity sizes according to sex were analyzed using the *t*-test, and differences in nasal cavity size according to FI and NI were analyzed using one-way analysis of variance and the post hoc Scheffe test. For all analyses, 95% confidence intervals (CI) are presented, and the significance level was set at 0.05.

3. Results

3.1. Nasal Dimensions According to Sex

Table 4 shows the differences in the nasal cavity sizes according to sex (Figure 7). The septum length of males was longer (75.72) than that of females (69.47) ($p < 0.001$). The septum height of males was higher (37.82) than that of females (37.53). However, the differences were not significant ($p > 0.05$). The length of the nasal cavities of males was higher (65.57) than that of females (56.64) ($p < 0.001$), and the height of the nasal cavities of males was higher (41.82) than that of females (40.51). However, the differences were not significant ($p > 0.05$).

Table 4. Nasal dimensions according to sex.

Parameter		N	Mean (SD)	F	T	p
Septum length	Male	50	75.72 (3.53)	0.085	9.278	0.000 *
	Female	50	69.47 (3.20)			
Septum height	Male	50	37.82 (5.48)	0.000	0.264	0.793
	Female	50	37.53 (5.46)			
Nasal cavity length	Male	50	65.57 (6.46)	0.001	6.864	0.000 *
	Female	50	56.64 (6.56)			
Nasal cavity height	Male	50	41.82 (6.15)	0.275	1.031	0.305
	Female	50	40.51 (6.53)			

Data are mean (standard-deviation values); p-values were obtained using t-tests (* $p < 0.001$).

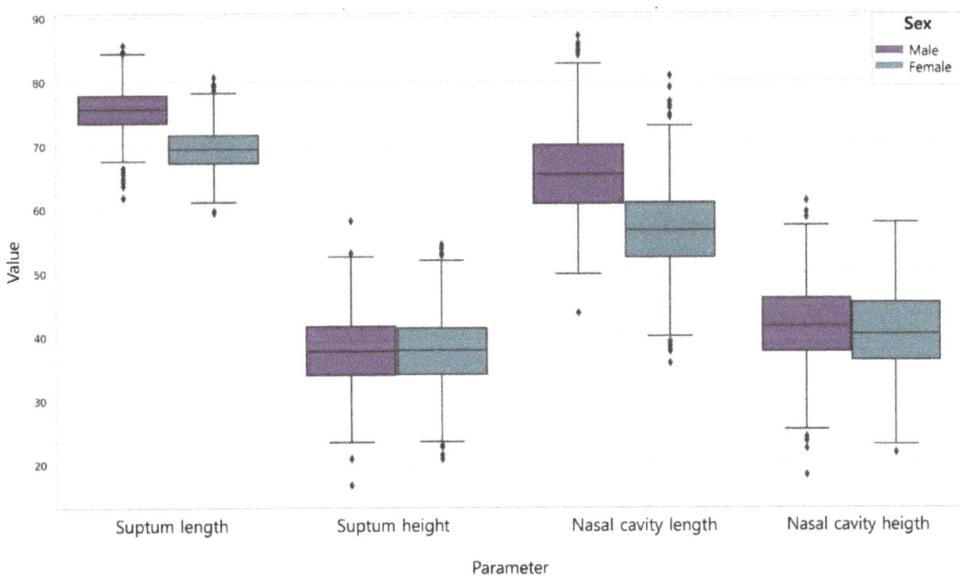

Figure 7. Nasal dimensions according to sex. Septum length was male > female ($p < 0.001$); septum height was male > female ($p > 0.05$). Nasal cavity length was male > female ($p < 0.001$); nasal cavity height was male > female ($p > 0.05$).

3.2. Nasal Dimensions According to the FI

Table 5 shows the differences in the nasal cavity sizes according to the FI (Figure 8). The septum length was longest for those with hypereuryprosopic (71.71), followed by euryprosopic (75.82) and mesoprosopic (72.95) facial shapes ($p < 0.001$). The septum height was highest for those with hypereuryprosopic (37.17), followed by euryprosopic (39.10) and mesoprosopic (39.49) facial shapes; however, the difference was not statistically significant ($p > 0.05$). The length of the nasal cavities was longest for those with hypereuryprosopic (59.74), followed by euryprosopic (65.89) and mesoprosopic (62.39) facial shapes ($p < 0.05$). The height of the nasal cavities was highest for those with hypereuryprosopic (41.05), followed by euryprosopic (40.79) and mesoprosopic (44.39) facial shapes; however, the difference was not statistically significant ($p > 0.05$).

Table 5. Nasal dimensions according to the FI.

Parameter		N	Mean (SD)	F	p
Septum length	Hypereuryprosopic	75	71.71 (4.47)	7.092	0.001 *
	Euryprosopic	20	75.82 (3.83)		
	Mesoprosopic	5	72.95 (4.14)		
Septum height	Hypereuryprosopic	75	37.17 (5.36)	1.285	0.281
	Euryprosopic	20	39.10 (5.70)		
	Mesoprosopic	5	39.49 (5.51)		
Nasal cavity length	Hypereuryprosopic	75	59.74 (7.53)	5.297	0.007 *
	Euryprosopic	20	65.89 (7.75)		
	Mesoprosopic	5	62.39 (7.25)		
Nasal Cavity height	Hypereuryprosopic	75	41.05 (6.55)	0.688	0.505
	Euryprosopic	20	40.79 (5.03)		
	Mesoprosopic	5	44.39 (8.21)		

Data are mean (standard-deviation values); p-values were obtained using one-way ANOVA (* $p < 0.001$).

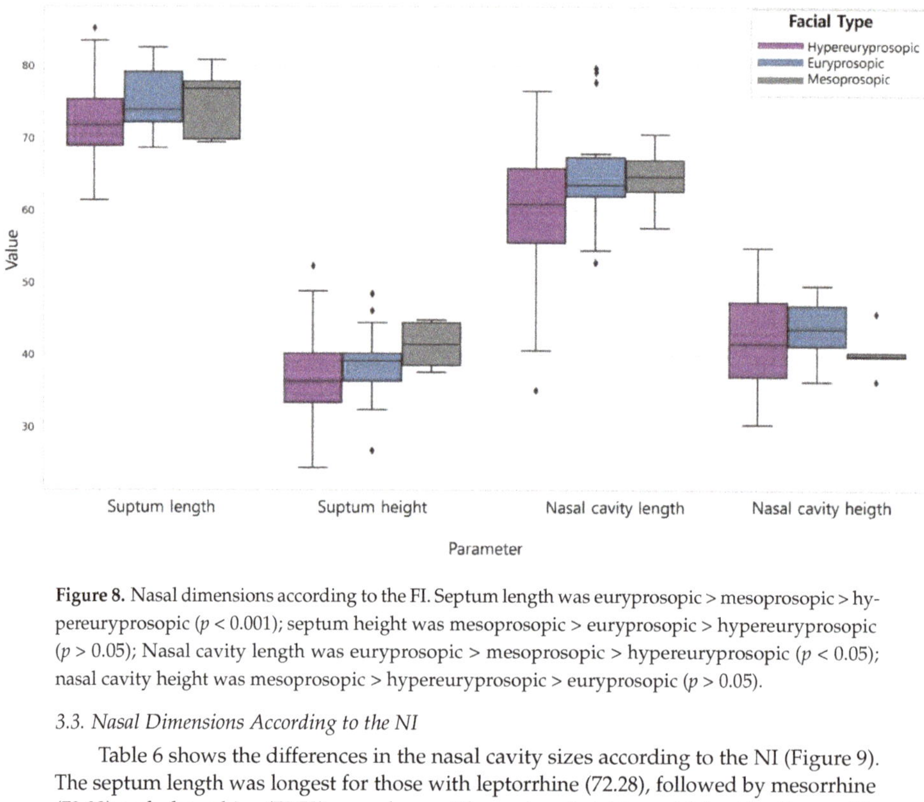

Figure 8. Nasal dimensions according to the FI. Septum length was euryprosopic > mesoprosopic > hypereuryprosopic ($p < 0.001$); septum height was mesoprosopic > euryprosopic > hypereuryprosopic ($p > 0.05$); Nasal cavity length was euryprosopic > mesoprosopic > hypereuryprosopic ($p < 0.05$); nasal cavity height was mesoprosopic > hypereuryprosopic > euryprosopic ($p > 0.05$).

3.3. Nasal Dimensions According to the NI

Table 6 shows the differences in the nasal cavity sizes according to the NI (Figure 9). The septum length was longest for those with leptorrhine (72.28), followed by mesorrhine (73.02) and platyrrhine (70.53) nose shapes. The septum height was highest for those with leptorrhine (39.93), followed by mesorrhine (37.46) and platyrrhine (37.22) nose shapes. The length of the nasal cavities was longest for those with leptorrhine (61.53), followed by mesorrhine (61.32) and platyrrhine (59.63) nose shapes. The length of the nasal cavities was highest for those with leptorrhine (39.71), followed by mesorrhine (41.83) and platyrrhine (38.60) nose shapes. However, the differences were not significant for any of them ($p > 0.05$).

Table 6. Nasal dimensions according to the NI.

Parameter		N	Mean (SD)	F	*p*
Septum length	Leptorrhine	10	72.28 (4.16)	1.792	0.172
	Mesorrhine	76	73.02 (3.77)		
	Platyrrhine	14	70.53 (3.77)		
Septum height	Leptorrhine	10	39.93 (3.95)	0.964	0.385
	Mesorrhine	76	37.46 (5.69)		
	Platyrrhine	14	37.22 (4.93)		
Nasal cavity length	Leptorrhine	10	61.53 (7.77)	0.284	0.753
	Mesorrhine	76	61.32 (8.41)		
	Platyrrhine	14	59.63 (4.56)		
Nasal cavity height	Leptorrhine	10	39.71 (5.56)	1.861	0.161
	Mesorrhine	76	41.83 (6.57)		
	Platyrrhine	14	38.60 (4.96)		

Data are mean (standard-deviation values); *p*-values were obtained using one-way ANOVA (* $p < 0.001$).

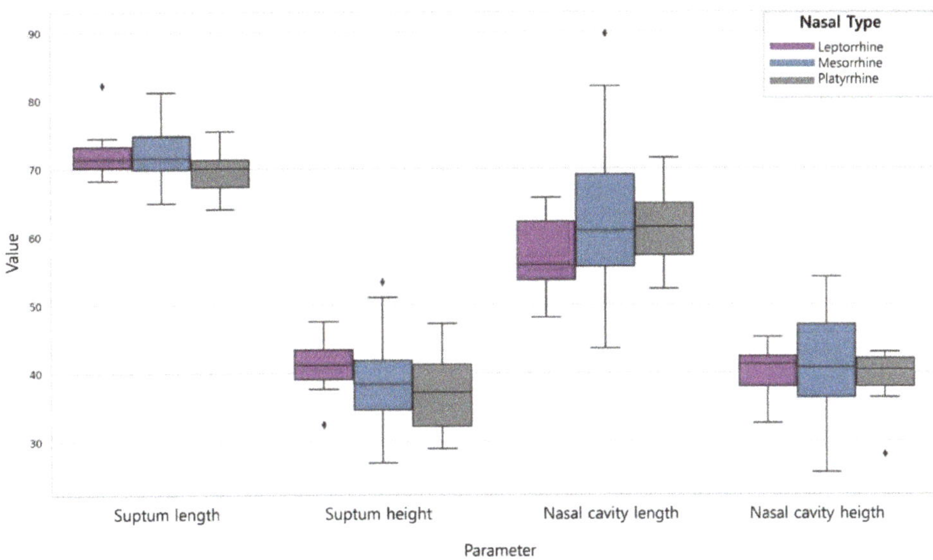

Figure 9. Nasal dimensions according to the NI. Septum length was mesorrhine > leptorrhine > platyrrhine ($p > 0.05$); septum height was leptorrhine > mesorrhine > platyrrhine ($p > 0.05$); nasal cavity length was leptorrhine > mesorrhine > platyrrhine ($p > 0.05$); nasal cavity height was mesorrhine > leptorrhine > platyrrhine ($p > 0.05$).

4. Discussion

The shape of the nasal cavity holds significant value not only in clinical contexts but also in forensic science [30]. However, the majority of morphometric studies have primarily focused on sex comparisons [1–14,19–38]. Therefore, it is necessary to examine how the nasal dimensions relate to the facial and nose dimensions. In this study, we aimed to anthropometrically compare nasal cavities based on sex, FI, and NI. FI and NI classifications were performed using 3D modeling.

The following results were obtained for the differences in nasal cavity size according to sex. The values of the septum length and height, and nasal cavity length and height of males were higher than that of females on average, similar to previous study findings [31,32]. Samoliński et al. [33] reported that the nasal cavity size varies across ages, sexes, and races. In addition, LoMauro et al. [34] reported that males have larger lungs and longer chest walls and diaphragms than females. Hence, males seem to have larger nasal cavities, which are influenced by the environment and climate. Thus, further research on sex-specific respiration and special considerations in clinical practice must be conducted.

The following results were obtained for the comparison of nasal cavity sizes according to the FI. Individuals with a broader or "euryprosopic" facial type had longer septum lengths, while those with a rounder or "mesoprosopic" facial type had higher septum heights. Additionally, the length of the nasal cavity was greater in individuals with a broader, euryprosopic facial type, while the height was greater in those with a rounder, mesoprosopic facial type. Thus, euryprosopic types generally tend to have a wider dimension, whereas mesoprosopic types tend to have taller dimensions. According to Butaric et al. [35], there may be potential variations in nasal cavity due to skull size and ecological characteristics. Hence, we were able to confirm that the facial skeletal structure influences the nasal cavity, highlighting the need for special considerations in clinical practice for nose-related care and research in forensic medicine.

The following results were obtained for the comparison of nasal cavity sizes according to the NI. The septum length was greater in the typical mesorrhine type, while height was greater in the elongated and narrow leptorrhine type. The length of the nasal cavity was greater in the elongated and narrow leptorrhine type, while height was greater in the typical mesorrhine type. Tomkinson et al. [36] compared the nasal cavity according to individual characteristics, such as height, weight, and facial width, and reported that the alar width is correlated with the size of the nasal cavity. We also observed that the nasal cavity size differs according to the nasal shape. Furthermore, Leong et al. [37] reported that the external proportions of the nose may be altered by physiological processes involving the internal structures. Therefore, nasal proportions should be considered when conducting nose-related research and clinical surgeries.

This study has the following limitations. Although there were differences in the mean measurements of nasal cavity sizes according to sex, FI, and NI, the differences were not statistically significant. Maddux et al. [38] reported that the inner structure of the nasal cavity is dependent on climate. Further, the nose is longer and larger relative to the cranium in cold and dry environments than that in hot and humid environments. This may be the reason underlying the lack of significant results in the differences in nasal cavity size according to sex, FI, and NI. Therefore, further research is needed to investigate nasal cavity sizes in relation to various factors and dimensions other than sex and skeletal dimensions, in consideration of the climate and environment.

In this study, we leveraged 3D modeling techniques to observe differences in nasal cavity sizes in relation to sex, FI, and NI. These findings are interpreted as indicative of the relationship between the structure of the nose and facial morphology and are deemed to hold significant implications for future research in the fields of forensic science and clinical practice. In the clinical domain, understanding the variations in nasal cavity sizes according to FI and NI indices could facilitate clinical diagnoses and surgical procedures. Specifically, this knowledge can be instrumental in planning surgeries for conditions requiring personalized treatment plans, such as nasal obstruction and obstructive sleep apnea, by considering the structure of the nose and individual anatomical differences. Consequently, this can aid in surgical outcomes for rhinoplasty and facial reconstruction surgeries, ultimately minimizing post-surgical complications, enhancing respiratory function and aesthetic results, and improving patient satisfaction and quality of life.

The results of this study have illustrated variability among groups by comparing nasal cavity sizes across genders, as well as FI and NI indices. This variability can be utilized to refine methods used in forensic anthropology for skull analysis, providing a more nuanced approach to the identification process. For instance, measurements of the nasal cavity dimensions could be associated with specific population groups when unidentified human remains are discovered, significantly improving the success rate of personal identification. Therefore, the outcomes derived from the anthropometric assessment using 3D modeling in this study are expected to benefit forensic practitioners in their tasks.

5. Conclusions

The findings of this study showed that nasal cavity sizes generally differed according to sex, FI, and NI. These results are expected to establish a crucial basis for the enhancement of tailored approaches within the realms of forensic and clinical medicine. Furthermore, this investigation has elucidated the substantial impact that anatomical variations within the nasal cavity may hold in both clinical and forensic settings, thereby underscoring the necessity for additional exploratory efforts concerning the nasal cavity. Importantly, it is anticipated that our findings will serve as foundational data for subsequent studies examining how the structural attributes of the nasal cavity are modulated by external environmental factors, such as the climate.

Author Contributions: Conceptualization, J.-H.L. and J.-T.P.; formal analysis, J.-H.L. and J.-T.P.; data curation, H.-S.K., J.-H.L. and J.-T.P.; writing—original draft preparation, H.-S.K., J.-H.L. and J.-T.P.; writing—review and editing, J.-H.L. and J.-T.P. All authors have read and agreed to the published version of the manuscript.

Funding: This study was supported by MRC (2021R1A5A2022318).

Institutional Review Board Statement: Ethical approval for this study was obtained from the institutional review board (DKUDH IRB 2020-01-007) of Dankook University Dental Hospital.

Informed Consent Statement: Informed consent was obtained from all subjects involved in the study.

Data Availability Statement: Original data are available upon request to the corresponding author.

Acknowledgments: The authors gratefully acknowledge the CBCT data support of Won-Jeong Han.

Conflicts of Interest: The authors declare no conflicts of interest.

References

1. Tian, L.; Dong, J.; Shang, Y.; Tu, J. Detailed comparison of anatomy and airflow dynamics in human and cynomolgus monkey nasal cavity. *Comput. Biol. Med.* **2022**, *141*, 105150. [CrossRef] [PubMed]
2. Im, S.; Heo, G.E.; Jeon, Y.J.; Sung, H.J.; Kim, S.K. Tomographic PIV measurements of flow patterns in a nasal cavity with geometry acquisition. *Exp. Fluids* **2014**, *55*, 1644. [CrossRef]
3. Luo, H.; Wang, J.; Zhang, S.; Mi, C. The application of frontal sinus index and frontal sinus area in sex estimation based on lateral cephalograms among Han nationality adults in Xinjiang. *J. Forensic Leg. Med.* **2018**, *56*, 1–4. [CrossRef] [PubMed]
4. Wilkinson, C.M. Facial reconstruction—Anatomical art or artistic anatomy? *J. Anat.* **2010**, *216*, 235–250. [CrossRef] [PubMed]
5. Hsiao, J.H.; Cottrell, G. Two fixations suffice in face recognition. *Psychol. Sci.* **2008**, *19*, 998. [CrossRef] [PubMed]
6. Guyomarc'h, P.; Stephan, C.N. The validity of ear prediction guidelines used in facial approximation. *J. Forensic Sci.* **2012**, *57*, 1427–1441. [CrossRef] [PubMed]
7. Guyomarc'h, P.; Dutailly, B.; Charton, J.; Santos, F.; Desbarats, P.; Coqueugniot, H. Anthropological facial approximation in three dimensions (AFA 3D): Computer-assisted estimation of the facial morphology using geometric morphometrics. *J. Forensic Sci.* **2014**, *59*, 1502–1516. [CrossRef]
8. Stephan, C.N. Facial approximation: An evaluation of mouth-width determination. *Am. J. Phys. Anthropol.* **2003**, *121*, 48–57. [CrossRef] [PubMed]
9. Rogers, T.L. Determining the sex of human remains through cranial morphology. *J. Forensic Sci.* **2005**, *50*, JFS2003385. [CrossRef]
10. Williams, B.A.; Rogers, T.L. Evaluating the accuracy and precision of cranial morphological traits for sex determination. *J. Forensic Sci.* **2006**, *51*, 729–735. [CrossRef]
11. Krishan, K.; Chatterjee, P.M.; Kanchan, T.; Kaur, S.; Baryah, N.; Singh, R.K. A review of sex estimation techniques during examination of skeletal remains in forensic anthropology casework. *Forensic Sci. Int.* **2016**, *261*, 165-e1. [CrossRef] [PubMed]
12. Scendoni, R.; Kelmendi, J.; Arrais Ribeiro, I.L.; Cingolani, M.; De Micco, F.; Cameriere, R. Anthropometric analysis of orbital and nasal parameters for sexual dimorphism: New anatomical evidences in the field of personal identification through a retrospective observational study. *PLoS ONE* **2023**, *18*, e0284219. [CrossRef] [PubMed]
13. Chen, F.; Chen, Y.; Yu, Y.; Qiang, Y.; Liu, M.; Fulton, D.; Chen, T. Age and sex related measurement of craniofacial soft tissue thickness and nasal profile in the Chinese population. *Forensic Sci. Int.* **2011**, *212*, 272-e1. [CrossRef] [PubMed]
14. Lee, U.Y.; Kim, H.; Song, J.K.; Kim, D.H.; Ahn, K.J.; Kim, Y.S. Assessment of nasal profiles for forensic facial approximation in a modern Korean population of known age and sex. *Leg. Med.* **2020**, *42*, 101646. [CrossRef] [PubMed]
15. Jayakrishnan, J.M.; Reddy, J.; Kumar, R.V. Role of forensic odontology and anthropology in the identification of human remains. *J. Oral Maxillofac. Pathol.* **2021**, *25*, 543–547. [CrossRef] [PubMed]

16. Akbar, A.; Chatra, L.; Shenai, P.K.; VeenaK, M.; Prabhu, R.V.; Shetty, P. Dental age estimation by pulp/tooth volume ratio based on cbct tooth images: A forensic study. *Indian J. Med. Res.* **2018**, *7*. Available online: https://www.worldwidejournals.com/paripex/article/dental-age-estimation-by-pulp-tooth-volume-ratio-based-on-cbct-tooth-images-a-forensic-study/ODU5NQ==/?is=1 (accessed on 1 April 2024). [CrossRef]
17. Sujatha, S.; Azmi, S.R.; Devi, B.K.; Shwetha, V.; Kumar, T.P. CBCT-the newfangled in forensic radiology. *J. Dent. Orofac. Res.* **2017**, *13*, 47–55.
18. Denny, C.; Bhoraskar, M.; Shaikh, S.A.A.; Bastian, T.S.; Sujir, N.; Natarajan, S. Investigating the link between frontal sinus morphology and craniofacial characteristics with sex: A 3D CBCT study on the South Indian population. *F1000Research* **2023**, *12*, 811. [CrossRef] [PubMed]
19. Doni, R.P.; Janaki, C.S.; Vijayaraghavan, V.; Raj, U.D. A study on measurement and correlation of cephalic and facial indices in male of South Indian population. *Int. J. Med. Res. Health Sci.* **2013**, *2*, 439–446.
20. Trivedi, H.; Azam, A.; Tandon, R.; Chandra, P.; Kulshrestha, R.; Gupta, A. Correlation between morphological facial index and canine relationship in adults—An anthropometric study. *J. Orofac. Sci.* **2017**, *9*, 16. [CrossRef]
21. Maalman, R.S.E.; Abaidoo, C.S.; Darko, N.D.; Tetteh, J. Facial types and morphology: A study among Sisaala and Dagaaba adult population in the Upper West Region, Ghana. *Sci. Afr.* **2019**, *3*, e00071. [CrossRef]
22. Porter, J.P.; Olson, K.L. Analysis of the African American female nose. *Plast. Reconstr. Surg.* **2003**, *111*, 627–628. [CrossRef]
23. Mehlum, C.S.; Rosenberg, T.; Dyrvig, A.K.; Groentved, A.M.; Kjaergaard, T.; Godballe, C. Can the Ni classification of vessels predict neoplasia? A systematic review and meta-analysis. *Laryngoscope* **2018**, *128*, 168–176. [CrossRef] [PubMed]
24. Alex, F.R.; Steven, B.; Timothy, G.L. *Human Body Composition*, 4th ed.; Human Kinetics Publishers: Champaign, IL, USA, 1996; pp. 167–172.
25. Olotu, J.E.; Eroje, A.; Oladipo, G.S.; Ezon-Ebidor, E. Anthropometric study of the facial and nasal length of adult Igbo ethnic group in Nigeria. *Int. J. Biol. Anthropol.* **2009**, *2*, 10–15.
26. Esomonu, U.G.; Ude, R.A.; Lukpata, P.U.; Nandi, E.M. Anthropometric study of the nasal index of Bekwara ethnic group of Cross River state, Nigeria. *Int. Res. J. Appl. Basic. Sci.* **2013**, *5*, 1262–1265.
27. Peter, F.; Jorgen, T.J. *Anatomy in Diagnostic Imaging*; Blackwell: Copenhagen, Denmark, 2001; pp. 22–24.
28. Pandeya, A.; Atreya, A. Variations in the facial dimensions and face types among the students of a Medical College. *JNMA J. Nepal Med. Assoc.* **2018**, *56*, 531. [CrossRef]
29. Milanifard, M.; Hassanzadeha, G. Anthropometric study of nasal index in Hausa ethnic population of northwestern Nigeria. *J. Contemp. Med. Sci.* **2018**, *4*, 26–29.
30. Liu, Y.; Johnson, M.R.; Matida, E.A.; Kherani, S.; Marsan, J. Creation of a standardized geometry of the human nasal cavity. *J. Appl. Physiol.* **2009**, *106*, 784–795. [CrossRef]
31. Russel, S.M.; Frank-Ito, D.O. Gender differences in nasal anatomy and function among Caucasians. *Facial Plast. Surg.* **2023**, *25*, 145–152. [CrossRef]
32. Wang, J.J.; Chiang, Y.F.; Jiang, R.S. Influence of Age and Gender on Nasal Airway Patency as Measured by Active Anterior Rhinomanometry and Acoustic Rhinometry. *Diagnostics* **2023**, *13*, 1235. [CrossRef]
33. Samoliński, B.K.; Grzanka, A.; Gotlib, T. Changes in nasal cavity dimensions in children and adults by gender and age. *Laryngoscope* **2007**, *117*, 1429–1433. [CrossRef] [PubMed]
34. LoMauro, A.; Aliverti, A. Sex differences in respiratory function. *Breathe* **2018**, *14*, 131–140. [CrossRef] [PubMed]
35. Butaric, L.N.; McCarthy, R.C.; Broadfield, D.C. A preliminary 3D computed tomography study of the human maxillary sinus and nasal cavity. *Am. J. Biol. Anthropol.* **2010**, *143*, 426–436. [CrossRef] [PubMed]
36. Tomkinson, A.; Eccles, R. External facial dimensions and minimum nasal cross-sectional area. *Clin. Otolaryngol.* **1995**, *20*, 557–560. [CrossRef] [PubMed]
37. Leong, S.C.; Eccles, R. A systematic review of the nasal index and the significance of the shape and size of the nose in rhinology. *Clin. Otolaryngol.* **2009**, *34*, 191–198. [CrossRef]
38. Maddux, S.D.; Butaric, L.N.; Yokley, T.R.; Franciscus, R.G. Ecogeographic variation across morphofunctional units of the humannose. *Am. J. Biol. Anthropol.* **2017**, *162*, 103–119. [CrossRef]

Journal of *Personalized Medicine*

MDPI

Article

Assessment of a New Medical Device (Pirifix^{TM}) for Positioning and Maintaining the Upper Dental Arch during Le Fort I Osteotomy

Pierre-Etienne Serree [1,2,*], Eugénie Bertin [1,2], Camille Coussens [2,3], Eleonore Brumpt [1,2,4], Jean-François Devoti [5] and Aurélien Louvrier [1,2,3]

1 Chirurgie Maxillo-Faciale, Stomatologie et Odontologie Hospitalière, CHU Besançon, Université de Franche-Comté, F-25000 Besançon, France; ebertin@chu-besancon.fr (E.B.); ebrumpt@chu-besancon.fr (E.B.); alouvrier@chu-besancon.fr (A.L.)
2 SINERGIES, Université de Franche-Comté, F-25000 Besançon, France; ccoussens@chu-besancon.fr
3 Plateforme I3DM (Impression 3D Médicale), CHU Besançon, Université de Franche-Comté, F-25000 Besançon, France
4 CHU Besançon, Radiologie, Université de Franche-Comté, F-25000 Besançon, France
5 Service de Chirurgie Maxillo-Faciale, Plastique, Reconstructrice et Esthétique, CHU Nancy, Université de Lorraine, F-54000 Nancy, France; j.devoti@chru-nancy.fr
* Correspondence: peserree@chu-besancon.fr; Tel.: +33-381668234

Abstract: Introduction: Several medical devices (MDs) are used to assist surgeons in positioning the upper dental arch (UDA) during Le Fort I osteotomies (LFIOs). Some only allow holding, others only positioning. This study aimed to assess the accuracy of a new MD (Pirifix^{TM}) coupling these two functions during LFIO on 3D-printed models. Materials and Methods: DICOM data were selected from patients who underwent surgical planning for LFIO between 27 July 2020 and 1 December 2022. Their anatomy was reproduced after segmentation, planning, and stereolithography in two models. Each model was assigned to one of two surgical groups: the control group (positioning by occlusal splint) and the Pirifix^{TM} group. Each patient's model was planned with the objective of horizontalizing and recentering the UDA. After positioning, models were digitalized using Einscan Pro 2X and compared to the planned model with CloudCompare. The statistical analysis was performed using the Wilcoxon Mann–Whitney test. The result was considered significant if the p-value was less than 0.05. Results: Twenty-one patients were selected. Forty-two anatomical models were 3D-printed. The mean difference compared to the planned and corrected positions was 0.69 mm for the control group and 0.84 mm for the Pirifix^{TM} group ($p = 0.036$). Conclusion: Pirifix^{TM} may be a new alternative to available MDs. Further investigations are needed to describe the relationship between the device and facial soft tissues.

Keywords: computer-aided design; equipment and supplies; orthognathic surgery; 3D printing

1. Introduction

Dentoskeletal disharmony is a frequent clinical condition whose etiology may be congenital or acquired. The description of the patient's facial morphology is based on clinical, 2D, and 3D radiological interpretation [1,2]. Orthognathic surgery complements orthodontics in the management of these disharmonies. It allows dental occlusion disorders to be corrected and aesthetic amelioration and orofacial functions to be improved. When the disharmony involves the maxillary bones, a Le Fort I osteotomy (LFIO) may be warranted. The correction of malposition is based on three axes of translation and three axes of rotation. Most often, it combines several movements, which makes positioning the maxillae more difficult [3,4].

Several medical devices (MDs) have been used for positioning the upper dental arch (UDA). These include occlusal splints, spacers [5,6], cutting guides combined with custom-made plates [7–15], and intraoperative navigation [10,16–20]. Each technique has limitations. Occlusal splints use a mobile bone, the mandible, as a reference for positioning the upper dental arch. Spacers only help surgeons with vertical dimensions without holding function. Custom-made plates are expensive and require a preoperative CT scan, which is associated with patient irradiation. Splints, guides, and custom-made plates are single-use medical devices with an environmental drawback. Intraoral navigation also requires preoperative planning and implies a specific installation in the operating theatre [16,21]. Furthermore, none of these devices allow for intraoperative adaptation in the same way as the mandibular on-site adjustment plates. All these devices are designed preoperatively and are not adjustable afterward. The assistance they provide becomes limited in complex cases of dentoskeletal disharmony requiring the surgeon to adapt the position of the upper dental arch intraoperatively. A medical device that combines support for the UDA with the ability for the operator to adjust its position would be ideal. The Ennoia company filed a patent in March 2023 for a new MD named Pirifix™, which meets these indications. It meets sterilizable class I MD defined by European regulations [22].

This study aimed to assess the precision of Pirifix™ for maintaining and adjusting the position of the upper dental arch during LFIO on models with dentoskeletal disharmony involving the middle third of the face.

2. Materials and Methods

2.1. Description of the Medical Device

The Pirifix™ device (Ennoïa, Besançon, France) is a bone-supported medical device. Its design is intended to adapt to the anatomy of the perimeter of the lower part of the piriform orifice (Figure 1). It is made up of ten parts produced in biocompatible 17-4ph stainless steel by selective laser melting technology. From top to bottom, the device consists of two paranasal bone-supported parts (right and left), which are associated with two vertical axes (right and left) and articulated with two anteroposterior axes (right and left) joined by a transverse axis (odd and median). This axis is also articulated at its center with an inverted U-shaped arch, with an inferior and posterior concavity. This arch carries the two premaxillary bone-supported parts (Figure 2). The device can be fixed on the skull with four screws (two below the line of an LFIO and two above). The various parts of the device are articulated together so that the palatal bone fragment can be moved in all three planes of space and then held in place. The two vertical axes are used for upward/downward and roll movements. The two anteroposterior axes are used for moving forward. An inverted U-shaped and the transversal axis allow for right or left translation and pitch. All the parts of the device are locked in the desired position by seven screws.

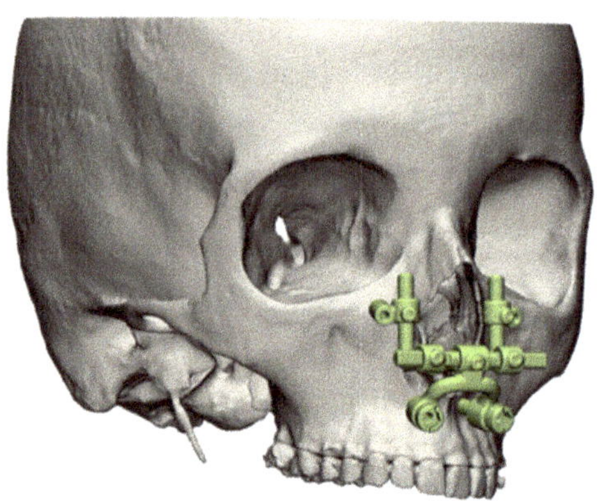

Figure 1. Three-dimensional illustration of Pirifix™ positioning around the piriform orifice.

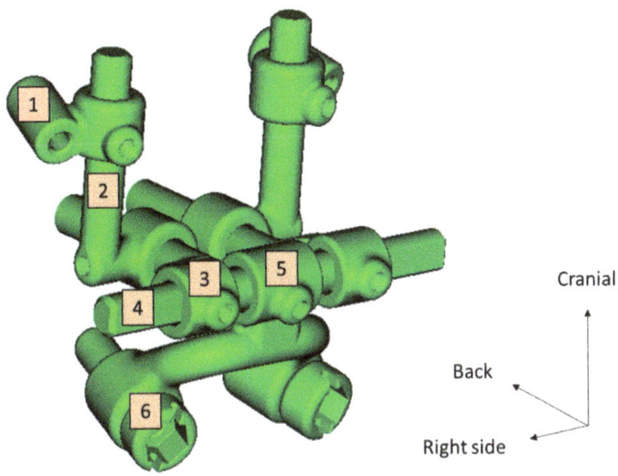

Figure 2. Experimental prototype file of Pirifix^{TM}. 1: Right paranasal bone support; 2: right vertical axis; 3: right anteroposterior axis; 4: transverse axis; 5: inverted U-shaped part; 6: right maxillary bone support.

2.2. *Creation of an Experimental Model*

2.2.1. Data Selection

DICOM data from patients who had virtual planned LFIOs between 27 July 2020 and 1 December 2022 were selected. This corresponds to all patient data archived at the Besançon University Hospital's 3D-printing platform since its inception. Exclusion criteria were the patient's opposition to the use of personal data, CT scans without all facial bones, CT scans with less than 300 slices, and no digital dental impression available. Ethical considerations, notably the absence of refusal by patients to use their data, were validated by the Clinical Research and Innovation Department of Besançon University Hospital. Sex, age at CT scan, Angle's classification and surgical treatments for each patient were noted to describe the population.

2.2.2. Conception

The models were designed and used on the Besançon University Hospital's 3D-printing platform. The procedure was repeated for each case included. Skulls and mandibles were segmented from DICOM data using Mimics Medical 25.0 software (Materialise, Leuven, Belgium). Corresponding dental models were added to the file. After a semi-automatic alignment step, segmented teeth were replaced by dental models. Alignment was considered complete when the average distance between the teeth from models and the segmented teeth on the CT scan was less than 0.01 mm.

Parts obtained in standard triangle language (STL) were then modified using 3-Matic 16.0 software (Materialise, Leuven, Belgium). Skull models were positioned on an orthogonal reference frame consisting of the median sagittal plane and the Frankfurt plane. The mandible was translated so far as to close the temporomandibular gap. Then, it was rotated clockwise around the bicondylar axe to remove overlapping between the mandibular and maxillary teeth. The calvaria was removed above a horizontal line passing through the middle of the forehead. The posterior part of the skull was removed behind a frontal plane passing between the foramen magnum and the mastoid processes. This plane was also used to develop a plate for fixing the skull to the table using a rail. An offset of 0.1 mm was applied to this rail, which was then subtracted from the skull by Boolean operation. The optic canals, orbital fissures, infraorbital foramina, and maxillary sinus were preserved. All other holes were filled. Skull surfaces were moderately smoothed.

Sixteen pairs of hooks were placed on each model. Six pairs reproduced orthodontic brackets. They were placed on the necks of the medial incisors, canines, and first premolars. Two pairs reproduced the resistance of the palatal mucosa. They were placed on the medial pterygoid processes and the posterior palate. Two pairs reproduced the temporomandibular joint capsule. They were placed on the base of the zygomatic arch and the condylar neck. Six pairs reproduced the muscular traction of the masseter, temporal, and medial pterygoid muscles. They were placed at their respective insertions (Figure 3).

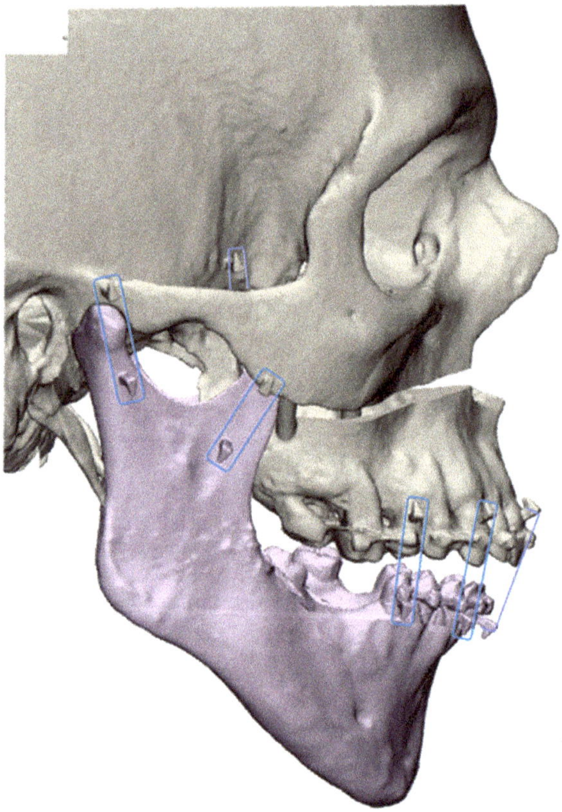

Figure 3. Example of an experimental model associating the mandible (in violet) with the rest of the skull. The pairs of hooks used to articulate the two objects are framed in blue.

LFIO and pterygopalatomaxillary disjunction (PPMD) were simulated using standardized boxes subtracted from the anatomical model. The LFIO box was herringbone-shaped and approximately 4 mm thick. It was centered on the midline. It cut through the vomer bone and maxillary sinus walls. Its posterior part was in continuity with the PPMD box. The PPMD box was a vertical 1 mm thick plane separating the pterygoid processes from the maxillary sinuses (Figure 4).

The models were completed by adding 4 cylindrical bridges between the UDA and the remaining skull. The right bridges were parallel to each other. The left bridges were also parallel. At the top, the bridges were supported on the internal cortical of the maxillary sinus lateral wall. At the bottom, they were supported on the maxillary sinus floor. The skulls with bridges and mandibles were recorded as two distinct objects for printing (Figure 5).

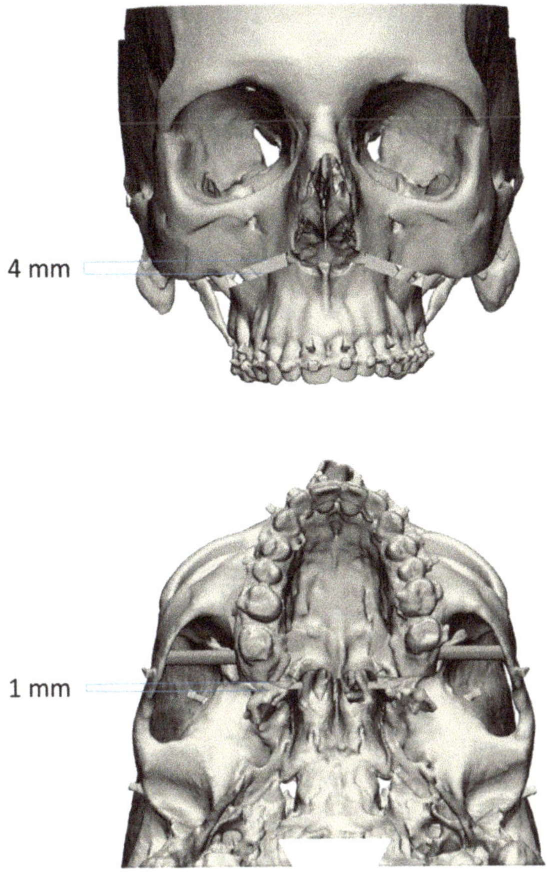

Figure 4. Example of an experimental model with Le Fort I osteotomy and pterygopalatomaxillary disjunction.

2.2.3. Planned Models

No modification of the UDA's position was applied to files used for printing. These files were also used as a reference to compare the return to the initial position (P0 position). To compare the groups in their ability to place the UDA in the corrected position (C position), a planned (reference) model was made for each patient. With these models, the UDA was horizontalized parallel to the Frankfurt plane. The interincisal point was centered on the median sagittal plane. For each planned model, the distance between the hooks of teeth 13 and 23 and the lowest point of the right and left infraorbital rims was recorded.

2.2.4. Splint Design

For each planned model, an occlusal positioning splint was designed using 3-Matic software. The upper and lower dental arches were circumscribed by a curve using a computer tool. The two curves were converted into a surface, and the space between these two surfaces was filled by constructing a three-dimensional object. An offset of 0.20 mm was applied to the dental arch models before being subtracted from the object by Boolean operation. The result was an arch-shaped splint bearing the maxillary and mandibular dental impressions in the planned position. It was used for P0 positioning (P0 splint) and C positioning (C splint).

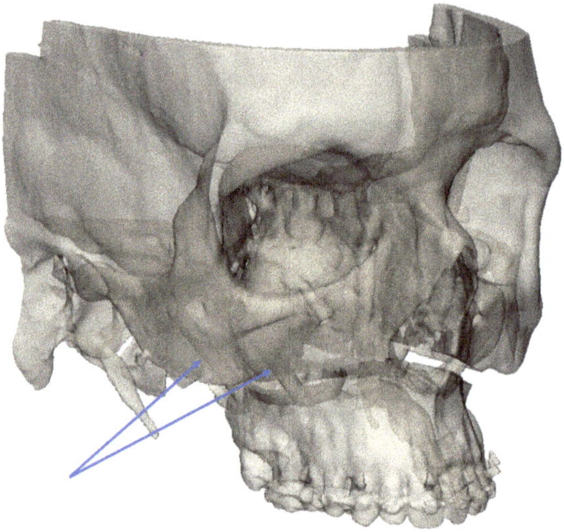

Figure 5. Example of experimental model seen in semi-transparency, showing the right bridges connecting the UDA to the rest of the skull (blue arrows).

2.2.5. Three-Dimensional Printing

Stereolithography was used with Preform software (Formlabs, Somerville, MA, USA) and a Form2 or Form3+ printer (Formlabs). The models were printed on a 1:1 scale with white resin (Figure 6), while the splints were printed with white, color base, or clear resin. The supports were manually removed. After, the models needed to be cleaned with a 20 min long isopropanol bath in FormWash (Formlabs) and they were then polymerized for 1 h with FormCure (Formlabs). Two copies of each model were printed. Each copy was assigned to one of two surgical groups: the control group (positioning by occlusal splint) and the Pirifix^{TM} group. The splints were printed using the same protocol as the experimental models and were assigned to the control group.

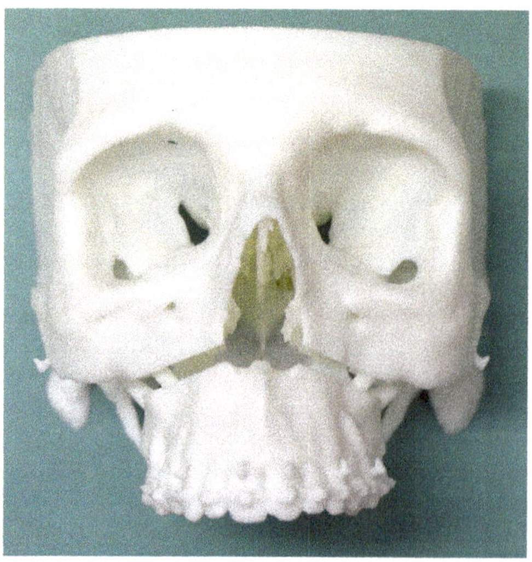

Figure 6. Example of an experimental 3D-printed model.

FDM technology was used to print fixation devices. The slicer software was Cura 4.6 and the printer was an Ultimaker 5 (Ultimaker, Utrecht, Netherlands).

2.2.6. Digitalizing

The models were scanned using an Einscan Pro 2x optical scanner (Shining 3D, Hangzhou, China). The angle between the rotative table and lens was 30°. We captured 30 shots per rotation. Four rotations were completed by changing the position of the models. During each 30 successive picture shot sequences, models were placed on the top edge, the back edge, the right temple, and the left temple. The watertight tool was turned off before making the mesh models. They were then cleaned up with 3-Matic by suppressing free voxels. Digitalizing was performed before UDA separation. After printing and before UDA separation, the printed models were digitalized for the first time and compared to the designed models to describe the printing and digitalizing precision and initial comparability of the groups.

2.2.7. Comparison

CloudCompare software (v2.13) was used to compare the models. First, they were manually superimposed. Next, we performed automatic matching between these two models based on the frontal, temporal, nasal, and zygomatic bones as the best overlapping areas (UDA segmented). This process was completed according to the root mean square setting at 1×10^{-7}. After matching, motion vectors were applied to the entire object comprising the UDA. Next, the digitalized models were segmented to only retain dental crowns. The surface was transformed into a cloud of one million points. We performed a cloud-to-mesh (C2M) comparison between the segmented cloud and the planned models as the reference. The absolute difference in millimeters and the standard deviation were noted.

2.3. *Evaluation of Device-Aided UDA Positioning Accuracy*

2.3.1. Positioning Procedure

The procedures were performed by only one junior surgeon. In the test group only, Pirifix™ was set, placed, and screwed around the piriform orifice before UDA separation. The screws used were 2 mm in diameter and 16 mm long for the upper fixings and 20 mm long for the lower fixings. Pirifix™ was then removed while maintaining the same setting.

Next, the connecting bridges were cut with pliers in each group. The mobile UDA and the mandible were attached to each skull using dental elastics (Southern Bald Eagle size ¼″ medium). The elastics were placed on hooks to reproduce muscular traction of the masseters, temporalis, medial pterygoid muscles, and palatine mucosa. The models were placed on the table using a fixing system.

Each UDA was then positioned according to the objectives set. Osteosynthesis was performed using modus 2 screws and titanium plates (Medartis, Basel, Switzerland). Positioning and osteosynthesis were performed twice per model. The first time, the UDA had to come back to its initial position. The second time, the UDA had to be positioned as the corrected and planned model. In each group, the vertical adjustment was set with a caliper in planned distances between the canine hooks and orbital rims.

In the control group, the first positioning was performed with a specific device. This one consisted of an initial position splint (P0 splint) and two spacers fitted into the osteotomy line. For the second positioning, we only used the occlusal splint (C splint) and the caliper.

In the test group, every positioning of the UDA was made only with Pirifix™ using holes around the piriform orifice. The P0 positioning was dictated by using the device without modifying the pre-separation setting. The C positioning was implemented by unlocking the vertical axes to adjust the tilt and impaction of the occlusal plane (Figure 7). In the Pirifix™ group, the osteosynthesis of the maxillo-zygomatic arches was performed first with Pirifix™ in place. Pirifix™ was then removed for paranasal osteosynthesis.

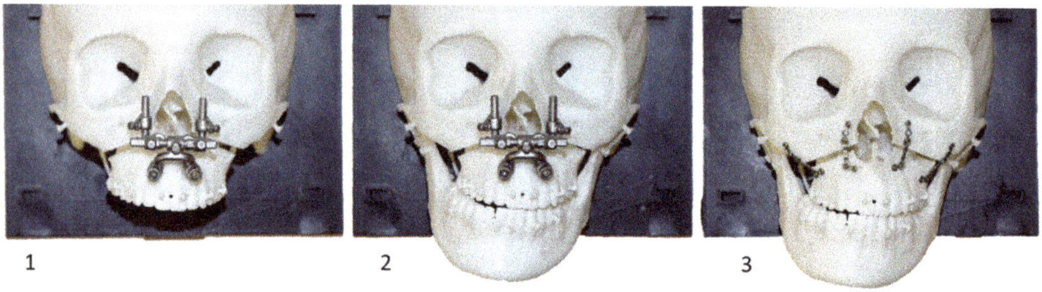

Figure 7. Operating procedure with Pirifix^{TM} (testing version) for movement C on model 14. 1: Repositioning of Pirifix^{TM}; 2: positioning of the UDA; 3: osteosynthesis (the two lateral plates before the removal of Pirifix^{TM}, the two medial plates after the removal of Pirifix^{TM}).

2.3.2. Digitalizing

After UDA separation and simulated surgery, the printed models of each group were digitalized for the second and the third time to be compared to the corresponding planned models (P0 movement and C movement, respectively). The digitalizing and comparison protocol applied to each model was the same for both groups.

2.3.3. Comparison of Precision

The accuracy of Pirifix^{TM} for placing the UDA in the planned and corrected positions was compared with the control group's efficiency. The visualization tool with the color scale of CloudCompare software was used to identify the areas where the difference was the most important. The vertical dimension included upward/downward and tilting movements. The horizontal dimension included lateral translation and horizontal rotation. The sagittal dimension included forward movements and clockwise/counterclockwise rotations.

2.4. Statistical Analysis

No data were available in the literature to estimate the expected difference in accuracy between Pirifix^{TM} and occlusal splints. The number of subjects required could not be determined. Data were analyzed using R statistical v4.2.2 (The R Foundation for Statistical Computing, Vienna, Austria). The mean difference between the models of the two groups and the planned models was compared. Analysis was performed by applying a Student's *t*-test or Wilcoxon Mann–Whitney test, depending on the number of models considered and variable distribution. Analyses were conducted as a two-sided test with 95% confidence intervals. The mean difference was considered significant if the *p*-value was less than 0.05.

3. Results

3.1. Experimental Models

Data from 21 patients were included (Figure 8). The characteristics of the population are described in Table 1. Twenty-one skulls were segmented from DICOM and then designed. Two copies of each model were printed and divided into two groups.

3.2. Assessment of Group Comparability before the Separation of the UDA

Each model in the two groups was digitalized after printing and before UDA separation and compared to the pre-printed files. The mean difference between the pre-printed files and the digitalized printed models was 0.19 mm (+/− 0.10) in the control group and 0.21 mm (+/− 0.09) in the Pirifix^{TM} group (p = 0.313).

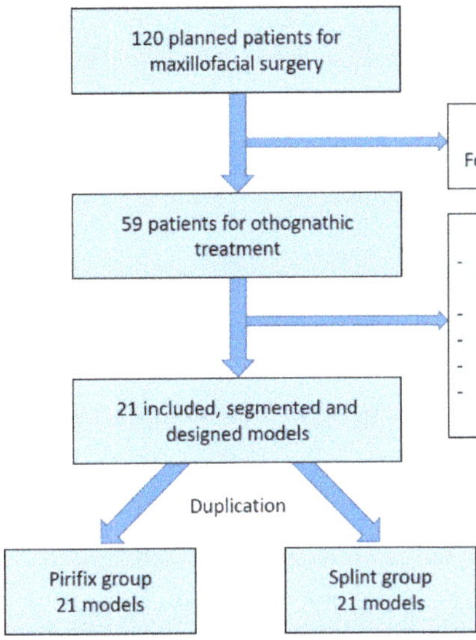

Figure 8. Flow chart. CT: computed tomography; BSSO: bilateral sagittal split osteotomy.

Table 1. Population characteristics. Yo: years old; LFIO: Le Fort I osteotomy; BSSO: bilateral sagittal split osteotomy.

Characteristics		Data
Sex		
	Female	15 (71.4%)
	Male	6 (28.6%)
Age		
	<20 yo	5 (23.8%)
	20 to 30 yo	8 (38.1%)
	30 to 40 yo	3 (14.3%)
	>40 yo	5 (23.8%)
	Average	28.6 yo (16 to 55)
Angle's classification		
	II	9 (42.9%)
	III	12 (57.1%)
Surgery		
	LFIO only	2 (9.5%)
	LFIO and BSSO	19 (90.5%)

3.3. Evaluation of Device-Aided UDA Positioning Accuracy

For the P0 position, the accuracy was 0.47 mm and 0.60 mm for the splint group and the Pirifix™ group, respectively (p = 0.054) (Figure 9). For the corrected position, the accuracy was 0.69 mm and 0.84 mm for the splint group and the Pirifix™ group, respectively (p = 0.036) (Figures 10 and 11). In the Pirifix™ for C positioning, 81.0% of models had an error in the vertical dimension, 61.9% in the sagittal dimension, and 66.7% in the horizontal dimension. In the splint group, this was 47.6%, 38.1%, and 76.2%, respectively.

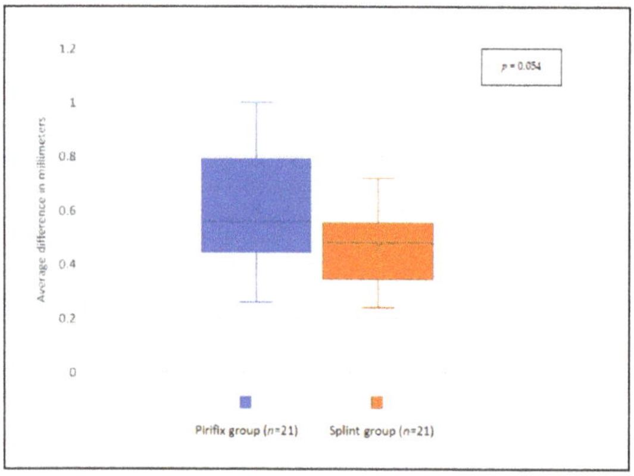

Figure 9. Comparison between planned files and printed models for P0 positioning in each group.

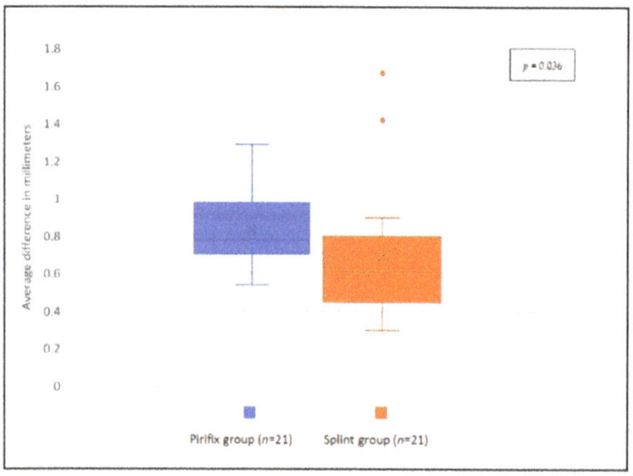

Figure 10. Comparison between planned files and printed models for C positioning in each group.

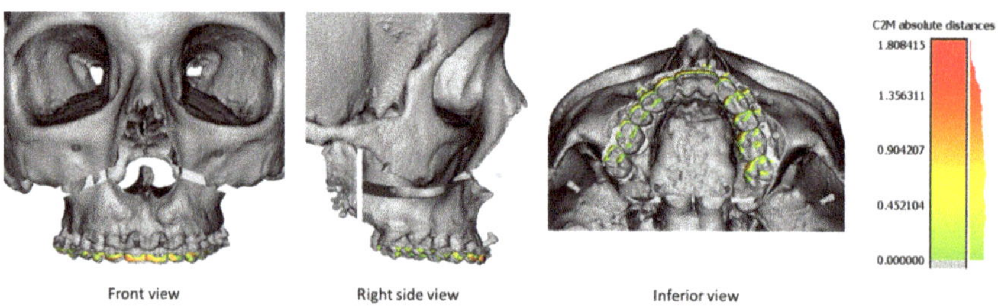

Figure 11. Superimposition between the 13 planned models (grey) and the 13 Pirifix^{TM}-positioned upper dental arches (color) for the P0 position. The color scale shows the difference in mm and the distribution of the difference.

4. Discussion

4.1. Experimental Models

The model's design meant that the osteotomy line had to be thick enough to perform rotational and translational movements without contact between the moving UDA and the upper osteotomy rim. The section was not intended to be a positioning guide.

The surface comparison of models was based on unmodified area matching. In their study describing a bone-and-teeth-supported surgical guide for LFIO, Kraeima et al. used zygomas, infraorbital margins, and foramen magnum [13]. Here, the UDA was subtracted from the model. The remaining file was also matched with the reference model. This provides a reliable assessment of the specific UDA-associated difference. Matching two whole objects would have superimposed them according to the smallest mean distance. In the event of an inhomogeneous difference, the difference would be smoothed over the entire model. This results in an increase in the observed difference of unmodified zones and an attenuation of the observed difference of zones that have been modified.

The comparability of both groups was ensured by the duplication of each model and their distribution in the two groups. Before the UDA's separation, the average difference compared with the pre-printed file was not significant between the two groups. Several hypotheses may explain the difference in variability observed from one model to another. It may be due to a different placement on the printing plate (dictated by the size of the model) or by the presence of movements of the printed model on the rotating plate of the optical scanner during digitalization.

4.2. Occlusal Splints

The 3D-printed occlusal splint was chosen as the reference method for two reasons. It remains a tried-and-tested method that has benefited from improved precision since 3D printing [10,23–25]. It is also less expensive and quicker to produce than custom-made titanium devices [14]. However, an occlusal splint is less accurate than surgical guides and custom-made osteosynthesis mesh [11,13,14].

4.3. Assessment of Pirifx^{TM}

For the P0 position, precision was not significantly better in the splint group than in the Pirifix^{TM} group. The inaccuracy observed in the control group for the P0 position may be the result of incorrect condylar positioning or the persistence of residual print supports in the spacer zone.

To prove the Pirifix^{TM} concept, we applied a movement combining horizontalizing and recentering the UDA. These movements were chosen for their larger aesthetic impact among both expert and non-expert observers [26]. For the C position, the accuracy of the UDA positioning performed by Pirifix^{TM} was significantly different from that of the splint group. The error observed in the splint group appears lower than in the Pirifix^{TM} group.

These results suggest that the difference associated with the use of Pirifix^{TM} is related more to the settings of the axes than to its paranasal repositioning.

The difference visualization tool with color scale showed that the difference in the splint group was predominantly in the horizontal dimension. In the Pirifix^{TM} group, the error was more a combination of inaccuracy in the three planes of space, but the vertical dimension was predominant. This result seems consistent insofar as Pirifix^{TM} is a standard device that can be adjusted in all planes. For the C position, Pirifix^{TM} essentially performed horizontalization. It may explain that the difference is more important in the vertical dimension. The splint, on the other hand, allows for positioning in the horizontal plane and frontal or sagittal tilting in the occlusal plane, without being able to set vertical translation. In this group, the difference was more important in the horizontal dimension. The condylar position can be responsible for diduction with rotation in the transverse plane. Insufficient posterior blocking may also be responsible for errors such as clockwise rotation. The use of the visualization tool described the difference in each dimension without specifying the amplitude of the error. On this point, the two groups are also not comparable.

In the Pirifix^{TM} group, positioning was assisted by the device but remained based on clinical criteria (only two measurements, assessment of centering and horizontalization). In addition, the device was fitted with clamping screws on a round-cut shaft, which could adversely affect the quality of locking. These factors may have influenced the results obtained in this group. The use of additional measures could improve the precision of the device. Furthermore, the models reproduced only the patient's bone, whereas facial symmetry is influenced by facial soft tissue in clinical practice.

The adaptability of Pirifix^{TM} was judged on the 21 included patients who had benefited from preoperative planning in the context of DSDy involving the midface. It was considered to have been achieved insofar as the adjustment of the device allowed for paranasal positioning without any identified conflicts. No bone conflicts were identified with the use of the device. Despite the anatomical diversity of the models, the number of patients is not enough to extrapolate the results to all midface disharmonies.

Among the MDs used for LFIO, Pirifix^{TM} offers a precise positioning alternative with a holding function that simplifies osteosynthesis. The splint allows for positioning in space with an error linked to a lack of predictability and reproducibility of the mandibular position. It can be used to adjust a tilt with an asymmetric thickness, but it cannot be used to adjust an upward or downward movement. These movements are associated with counterclockwise and clockwise rotation, respectively, due to mandibular rotation. The Pirifix^{TM} device is not custom-made and therefore has lower theoretical accuracy. However, it is supported on fixed bones above the osteotomy. This makes it more predictable, with a final inaccuracy of around 0.84 mm. The question arises as to the clinical relevance of precision in this context. Correct positioning must also be judged in terms of aesthetic consistency, involving facial soft tissues, and integration into the orthodontist's treatment plan.

The control group models were printed and operated on first. The results may be influenced by the learning process of the operator. This would apply in the handling of the caliper and the intraoperative taking of clinical measurements. All the models were operated on by a single surgeon. Feedback from many operators is needed to define the limits and improve the ergonomics of the device. A measurement bias is possible because the operator necessarily knows which device they have used for positioning. This bias was reproduced during the digitization and comparison phase since the same investigator was involved.

This is a preliminary study carried out on a 3D-printed simulator with no soft tissue. The aim was to prove the concept of this new medical device. Further investigations are still required, including facial soft tissue and technical feedback from other surgeons. The biocompatibility of the MD will have to be qualified before considering clinical trials. Pirifix^{TM} claims need to be assessed in studies conducted in clinical practice. The device is designed to simplify the positioning and maintaining of the UDA in the desired position during osteosynthesis. Its intraoperative adaptability makes it an attractive alternative to devices such as occlusal splints or custom plates. It remains to be seen how satisfactory the postoperative functional and aesthetic results will be. The invasiveness of the device, particularly when screwed around the piriform orifice, has yet to be assessed. The design of the lower parts seeks to avoid damaging the dental apexes. However, the design of the upper supports exposes patients to the risk of injury to the nasolacrimal ducts. Finally, the indications for its use need to be defined for a range of more or less complex disharmonies.

5. Conclusions

Pirifix^{TM} is a new medical device. It is positioned as an alternative to other medical devices for positioning the upper dental arch during LFIO. It also claims to have a holding function to facilitate fixation. The Pirifix^{TM} concept seems to be producing encouraging results. There are many ways of optimizing the process by modifying design or production technology. The architecture of the device could make it possible to dissociate each translation and rotation movement. All parts could be miniaturized to reduce the overall dimensions. The use of Pirifix^{TM} for complex movements combining more than one rotation and one translation has yet to be investigated. Further studies are needed to determine how the device works with other bone anatomies, as well as with soft tissues.

Author Contributions: Conceptualization, A.L. and P.-E.S.; methodology, A.L. and P.-E.S.; software, C.C.; validation, A.L.; data curation, P.-E.S., E.B. (Eugénie Bertin), E.B. (Eléonore Brumpt), and J.-F.D.; writing—original draft preparation, P.-E.S.; writing—review and editing, A.L.; supervision, A.L. All authors have read and agreed to the published version of the manuscript.

Funding: This research received no external funding.

Institutional Review Board Statement: Not applicable.

Informed Consent Statement: Not applicable.

Data Availability Statement: Data are contained within the article.

Acknowledgments: The authors would like to thank Benjamin Billottet (Ennoïa, Besancon, France).

Conflicts of Interest: All authors declare that they have no conflicts of interest.

References

1. Lonic, D.; Pai, B.C.-J.; Yamaguchi, K.; Chortrakarnkij, P.; Lin, H.-H.; Lo, L.-J. Computer-Assisted Orthognathic Surgery for Patients with Cleft Lip/Palate: From Traditional Planning to Three-Dimensional Surgical Simulation. *PLoS ONE* **2016**, *11*, e0152014. [CrossRef] [PubMed]
2. Terajima, M.; Nakasima, A.; Aoki, Y.; Goto, T.K.; Tokumori, K.; Mori, N.; Hoshino, Y. A 3-dimensional method for analyzing the morphology of patients with maxillofacial deformities. *Am. J. Orthod. Dentofac. Orthop.* **2009**, *136*, 857–867. [CrossRef] [PubMed]
3. Béziat, J.-L. *Chirurgie Orthognathique Piézoélectrique*; EDP Sciences: Les Ulis, France, 2013; ISBN 978-2-7598-0650-8.
4. Mulier, D.; Shaheen, E.; Shujaat, S.; Fieuws, S.; Jacobs, R.; Politis, C. How accurate is digital-assisted Le Fort I maxillary osteotomy? A three-dimensional perspective. *Int. J. Oral Maxillofac. Surg.* **2020**, *49*, 69–74. [CrossRef] [PubMed]
5. Dumrongwongsiri, S.; Lin, H.-H.; Niu, L.-S.; Lo, L.-J. Customized Three-Dimensional Printing Spacers for Bone Positioning in Orthognathic Surgery for Correction and Prevention of Facial Asymmetry. *Plast. Reconstr. Surg.* **2019**, *144*, 246e–251e. [CrossRef]
6. Abu-Serriah, M.; Wong, L.; Saeed, N. Adjunct to intraoperative control of vertical movement in inferiorly positioned Le Fort I maxillary osteotomy. *Br. J. Oral Maxillofac. Surg.* **2017**, *55*, 222–223. [CrossRef]
7. Huang, S.-F.; Lo, L.-J.; Lin, C.-L. Biomechanical optimization of a custom-made positioning and fixing bone plate for Le Fort I osteotomy by finite element analysis. *Comput. Biol. Med.* **2016**, *68*, 49–56. [CrossRef]
8. Wong, A.; Goonewardene, M.S.; Allan, B.P.; Mian, A.S.; Rea, A. Accuracy of maxillary repositioning surgery using CAD/CAM customized surgical guides and fixation plates. *Int. J. Oral Maxillofac. Surg.* **2021**, *50*, 494–500. [CrossRef]
9. Tankersley, A.C.; Nimmich, M.C.; Battan, A.; Griggs, J.A.; Caloss, R. Comparison of the Planned Versus Actual Jaw Movement Using Splint-Based Virtual Surgical Planning: How Close Are We at Achieving the Planned Outcomes? *J. Oral Maxillofac. Surg.* **2019**, *77*, 1675–1680. [CrossRef]
10. Lin, H.-H.; Lonic, D.; Lo, L.-J. 3D printing in orthognathic surgery—A literature review. *J. Formos. Med. Assoc.* **2018**, *117*, 547–558. [CrossRef]
11. Kraeima, J.; Schepers, R.H.; Spijkervet, F.K.L.; Maal, T.J.J.; Baan, F.; Witjes, M.J.H.; Jansma, J. Splintless surgery using patient-specific osteosynthesis in Le Fort I osteotomies: A randomized controlled multi-centre trial. *Int. J. Oral Maxillofac. Surg.* **2020**, *49*, 454–460. [CrossRef]
12. Suojanen, J.; Leikola, J.; Stoor, P. The use of patient-specific implants in orthognathic surgery: A series of 32 maxillary osteotomy patients. *J. Cranio-Maxillofac. Surg.* **2016**, *44*, 1913–1916. [CrossRef]
13. Kraeima, J.; Jansma, J.; Schepers, R.H. Splintless surgery: Does patient-specific CAD-CAM osteosynthesis improve accuracy of Le Fort I osteotomy? *Br. J. Oral Maxillofac. Surg.* **2016**, *54*, 1085–1089. [CrossRef] [PubMed]
14. Li, B.; Wei, H.; Jiang, T.; Qian, Y.; Zhang, T.; Yu, H.; Zhang, L.; Wang, X. Randomized Clinical Trial of the Accuracy of Patient-Specific Implants versus CAD/CAM Splints in Orthognathic Surgery. *Plast. Reconstr. Surg.* **2021**, *148*, 1101–1110. [CrossRef] [PubMed]
15. Chen, Z.; Mo, S.; Fan, X.; You, Y.; Ye, G.; Zhou, N. A Meta-analysis and Systematic Review Comparing the Effectiveness of Traditional and Virtual Surgical Planning for Orthognathic Surgery: Based on Randomized Clinical Trials. *J. Oral Maxillofac. Surg. Off. J. Am. Assoc. Oral Maxillofac. Surg.* **2021**, *79*, 471.e1–471.e19. [CrossRef]
16. Benassarou, M.; Benassarou, A.; Meyer, C. La navigation en chirurgie orthognathique. Application à l'ostéotomie de Le Fort I. *Rev. Stomatol. Chir. Maxillo-Faciale Chir. Orale* **2013**, *114*, 219–227. [CrossRef]
17. Lartizien, R.; Zaccaria, I.; Noyelles, L.; Bettega, G. Quantification of the inaccuracy of conventional articulator model surgery in Le Fort 1 osteotomy: Evaluation of 30 patients controlled by the Orthopilot® navigation system. *Br. J. Oral Maxillofac. Surg.* **2019**, *57*, 672–677. [CrossRef]
18. Lartizien, R.; Zaccaria, I.; Noyelles, L.; Bettega, G. Improvement in accuracy of maxillary repositioning of Le Fort I osteotomy with Orthopilot™ Navigation System: Evaluation of 30 patients. *Br. J. Oral Maxillofac. Surg.* **2020**, *58*, 1116–1122. [CrossRef]
19. Marmulla, R.; Mühling, J.; Lüth, T.; Hassfeld, S. Physiological shift of facial skin and its influence on the change in precision of computer-assisted surgery. *Br. J. Oral Maxillofac. Surg.* **2006**, *44*, 273–278. [CrossRef]

20. Sun, Y.; Luebbers, H.-T.; Agbaje, J.O.; Schepers, S.; Vrielinck, L.; Lambrichts, I.; Politis, C. Evaluation of 3 different registration techniques in image-guided bimaxillary surgery. *J. Craniofac. Surg.* **2013**, *24*, 1095–1099. [CrossRef]
21. Berger, M.; Nova, I.; Kallus, S.; Ristow, O.; Eisenmann, U.; Freudlsperger, C.; Seeberger, R.; Hoffmann, J.; Dickhaus, H. Electromagnetic navigated positioning of the maxilla after Le Fort I osteotomy in preclinical orthognathic surgery cases. *Oral Surg. Oral Med. Oral Pathol. Oral Radiol.* **2017**, *123*, 298–304. [CrossRef]
22. Le Parlement Européen et le Conseil de l'Union Européenne. Règlement (UE) 2017/745 du Parlement Européen et du Conseil—Du 5 avril 2017—Relatif aux dispositifs médicaux, modifiant la directive 2001/83/CE, le règlement (CE) no 178/2002 et le règlement (CE) no 1223/2009 et abrogeant les directives du conseil 90/385/CEE et 93/42/CEE. *J. Off. l'Union Eur.* **2017**, *117*, 175.
23. Lauren, M.; McIntyre, F. A new computer-assisted method for design and fabrication of occlusal splints. *Am. J. Orthod. Dentofac. Orthop.* **2008**, *133*, S130–S135. [CrossRef]
24. Shaheen, E.; Sun, Y.; Jacobs, R.; Politis, C. Three-dimensional printed final occlusal splint for orthognathic surgery: Design and validation. *Int. J. Oral Maxillofac. Surg.* **2017**, *46*, 67–71. [CrossRef]
25. Zinser, M.J.; Sailer, H.F.; Ritter, L.; Braumann, B.; Maegele, M.; Zöller, J.E. A paradigm shift in orthognathic surgery? A comparison of navigation, computer-aided designed/computer-aided manufactured splints, and "classic" intermaxillary splints to surgical transfer of virtual orthognathic planning. *J. Oral Maxillofac. Surg. Off. J. Am. Assoc. Oral Maxillofac. Surg.* **2013**, *71*, 2151.e1–2151.e21. [CrossRef] [PubMed]
26. Kokich, V.O.; Kiyak, H.A.; Shapiro, P.A. Comparing the perception of dentists and lay people to altered dental esthetics. *J. Esthet. Dent.* **1999**, *11*, 311–324. [CrossRef] [PubMed]

Journal of Personalized Medicine

MDPI

Article

Guided Genioplasty: Comparison between Conventional Technique and Customized Guided Surgery

Raúl Antúnez-Conde Hidalgo [1], José Luis Silva Canal [1], Carlos Navarro Cuéllar [2,3,*], Celia Sánchez Gallego-Albertos [1], Javier Arias Gallo [1], Ignacio Navarro Cuéllar [2], Antonio López Davis [1], Gastón Demaria Martínez [1], Néstor Naranjo Aspas [1], José Zamorano León [4] and Manuel Chamorro Pons [1]

1 Maxillofacial Surgery Department, Hospital Universitario Ruber Juan Bravo, 28006 Madrid, Spain; raul@antunezcondemaxilofacial.com (R.A.-C.H.); joseluis_silva92@hotmail.com (J.L.S.C.); drasanchezgallego@gmail.com (C.S.G.-A.); javierariasgallo@gmail.com (J.A.G.); alpzdvs@gmail.com (A.L.D.); gastondemaria@gmail.com (G.D.M.); nestornaranjo.lp@gmail.com (N.N.A.); mchamorropons@hotmail.com (M.C.P.)

2 Maxillofacial Surgery Department, Hospital General Universitario Gregorio Marañón, 28007 Madrid, Spain; ignacio.navarro@salud.madrid.org

3 Surgery Department, Universidad Complutense de Madrid, 28040 Madrid, Spain

4 Department of Public Health and Maternal and Child Health, Faculty of Medicine, Universidad Complutense de Madrid, 28040 Madrid, Spain; jjzamorano@ucm.es

* Correspondence: cnavarroc@salud.madrid.org

Abstract: Background: Genioplasty as an isolated surgical technique is a highly demanded procedure in the maxillofacial surgery area. Advances in facial reconstructive surgery have been associated with less morbidity and more predictable results. In this paper, "conventional" genioplasty and genioplasty by means of virtual surgical planning (VSP), CAD-CAM cutting guides, and patient custom-made plates are compared. Methods: A descriptive observational study was designed and implemented, and 43 patients were treated, differentiating two groups according to the technique: 18 patients were treated by conventional surgery, and 25 patients were treated through virtual surgical planning (VSP), CAD-CAM cutting guides, STL models, and titanium patient-specific plates. Results: The operation time ranged from 35 to 107 min. The mean operative time in the conventional group was 60.06 + 3.74 min.; in the custom treatment group it was 42.24 + 1.29 min ($p < 0.001$). The difference between planned and obtained chin changes in cases of advancement or retrusion was not statistically significant ($p = 0.125$; $p = 0.216$). In cases of chin rotation due to asymmetry, guided and personalized surgery was superior to conventional surgery ($p < 0.01$). The mean hospital stay was equal in both groups. A decrease in surgical complications was observed in the group undergoing VSP and customized treatment. Conclusions: Multi-stage implementation of VSP with CAD-CAM cutting guides, STL models, and patient-specific plates increased the accuracy of the genioplasty surgery, particularly in cases of chin asymmetry, reducing operation time and potential complications.

Keywords: genioplasty; chin deformity; virtual surgical planning; CAD-CAM technology; stereolithographic models; patient-specific plates; head and neck reconstruction; aesthetic surgery

1. Introduction

Genioplasty consists of an osteotomy of the anteroinferior border of the mandible, allowing movement of the chin in the three dimensions of space and placing it in the desired new position. It is a highly in-demand procedure in the context of maxillofacial and plastic surgery. The technique was described in the 19th century, and it became popular in the last decades of the 20th century as a complement to the surgical correction of dentofacial deformities [1,2]. Progressively, surgical techniques have been refined from aggressive osteotomies with wire-type fixations through alloplastic grafts to chin osteotomy with semi-rigid osteosynthesis for the correction of chin projection and/or asymmetry. The increase in social demand for correcting dental and/or skeletal problems and the greater coordination between orthodontists and maxillofacial surgeons have led to the standardization of this procedure, associated or not, with mono- or bimaxillary orthognathic surgery within the usual care activity of oral and maxillofacial surgery departments [2–5].

Advances in reconstructive surgical techniques in the head and neck area have allowed a comprehensive treatment and a complete surgical approach, with significant improvement in aesthetic and functional reconstruction, fewer comorbidities, and better recovery for the patients [6]. Less aggressive surgical techniques, additive manufacturing, and digital workflow have significantly improved comprehensive reconstruction of the facial skeleton [5–8], including surgical treatment of the chin. In this context, the development of virtual surgical planning (VSP), CAD-CAM technology, and the manufacture of cutting guides and customized titanium mini-plates have brought about a paradigm shift in the surgical treatment of mandibular deformities. Semi-rigid fixation for chin osteotomy is considered the main osteosynthesis technique, although traditionally, the material for bone fixation was not customized [9]. This study compares two genioplasty techniques: conventional genioplasty by osteotomy and semi-rigid fixation with screws and mini-plates with "freehand" planning, and genioplasty by osteotomy with customized cutting guides and personalized plates prior to VSP.

2. Materials and Methods

To address the research purpose, the authors designed and implemented a descriptive observational study with 43 patients diagnosed with chin deformity (excess, defect, or asymmetry) between 2019 and 2023 at the Hospital Universitario Ruber Juan Bravo, Madrid, Spain. Eighteen patients were treated by means of the conventional genioplasty technique with osteotomy and semi-rigid fixation with non-customized material. The remaining 25 patients underwent surgery after virtual surgical planning (VSP) design and manufacture of specific cutting guides and titanium plates using CAD-CAM technology. Patients treated with conventional surgery were treated between 2019 and 2021.

Inclusion criteria were: (1) patients with a diagnosis of chin deformity; (2) patients reconstructed with the "conventional" technique; and (3) patients treated with VSP, custom cutting guides, and titanium plates. Exclusion criteria were: (1) patients with previous surgery or surgical sequelae affecting the mandibular region. Follow-up ranged from 6 to 50 months.

This study followed the Declaration of Helsinki on medical protocol, and the study and review of medical records, data collection, and subsequent analysis are endorsed by the Hospital Ethics Committee (protocol code rjbmaxilo 01/2024).

In the cases treated by traditional methods, a preoperative CT scan was performed on all patients in DICOM format, which was subsequently edited with open-access software in order to obtain a stereolithographic model (STL) with 3D printing in polyamide. A "model surgery" was performed on this template in order to propose the most suitable surgical movements in each case and thus decide on the optimal positioning of the chin. The titanium plates adapted to the patient's anatomy were molded preoperatively. Once in the operating room, an intraoral approach was performed in all cases, identifying and preserving the chin nerves. The osteotomy line was marked, and the osteotomy was performed in the most appropriate region, taking into account the previous work on the 3D models. It was performed with a piezoelectric scalpel, and the fixation of the bone was made with mini-plates and titanium screws.

In cases treated through VSP, cutting guides, and patient-customized plates, a remote connection was established with the engineering team of the corresponding manufacturer (Avinent Implant System S.L.U, Santpedor, Barcelona, Spain). The osteotomy cutting guides were designed using CAD-CAM technology and produced with a 3D printer in polyamide; a surface and volumetric measurement of the chin positioning was performed on the virtual model once the osteotomy had been delimited, and a customized titanium prosthesis was designed for each patient. The customized titanium plates were fabricated using CAD-CAM technology, and they were manufactured with a DMG HSC (high-speed cutting) milling machine (Avinent Implant System S.L.U, Santpedor, Barcelona, Spain). Irregular edges or protrusions that could compromise the patient's comfort or aesthetic results were avoided. The optimal fit of the bone-cutting guides and the plates (Avinent Implant System S.L.U, Santpedor, Barcelona, Spain) was checked on printed STL models. An intraoral approach was performed in all cases. After identification and preservation of the mentonian nerves, the two-piece cutting guide was adapted, and the osteotomy was performed with a piezoelectric scalpel. The planned chin movement was performed, and semi-rigid osteosynthesis was effectuated with titanium plates and screws according to the manufacturer's instructions (Figure 1).

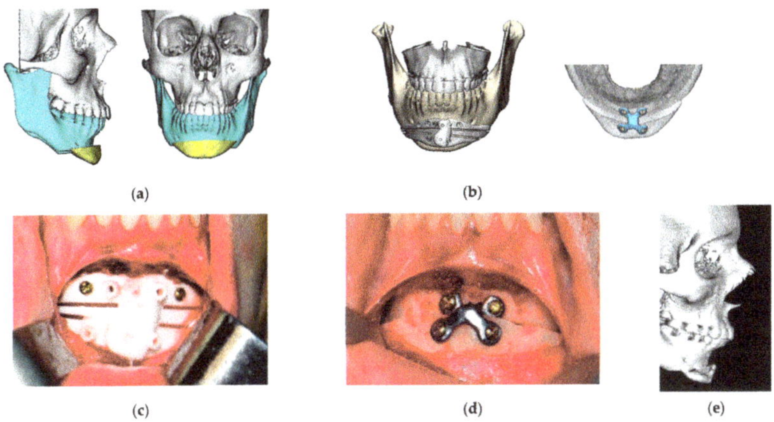

Figure 1. Customized guided surgery. (**a**) Virtual surgical planning and design of the osteotomy. Sagittal and front view; (**b**) digital design of cutting guide and titanium plate. Avinent Implant System S.L.U, Santpedor, Barcelona, Spain; (**c**) intraoperative photograph: fitting of cutting guide; (**d**) intraoperative photograph: final position of the chin with customized titanium plate and screws; (**e**) six-month post-operative control CT. Sagittal view.

All cases were also studied by preoperative and postoperative computed tomography (CT). Sagittal plane movement (advancement or retrusion) of the chin was measured in millimeters. In cases of asymmetry, chin rotation was measured in degrees, taking the nasion–chin vertical as a reference.

To generate the 3D anatomical model, the preoperative CT scan was obtained in DICOM format. The files were processed using the medical software Mimics Innovation© Suite 20.0. The virtual design of the sagittal movements of the chin was performed using Dolphin Imaging Software© (version 10.5, Canoga Park, CA, USA), modeling the target according to the patient's wishes and the experience of the surgical team. Before fabrication of the cutting guides and custom mini-plates, the virtual design of all the material was checked by the surgeon before approval or modification.

The operative time was also measured in all cases. Moreover, all patients were asked about their perception of the aesthetic result 6 months after surgery.

The variables evaluated in this study were:

(1) Difference between planned and achieved motion with both techniques (measured in millimeters, and in degrees for chin rotation cases). The Phillips IntelliSpace Portal© V.11.1(Koninklijke Philips N.V. Amsterdam, The Nederlands). radiological viewer was used for this purpose.
(2) Intervention time and length of hospital stay between the two techniques.
(3) Aesthetic outcome: an aesthetic assessment was performed by the patients to address scores in facial symmetry, facial healing, and facial projection. The results were classified as "excellent", "good", and "poor".

Statistical analysis was performed with SPSS© 28.0 software (IBM SPSS Statistics, Chicago, IL, USA).

3. Results

Forty-three patients were included in the study. Eighteen patients were treated by the conventional genioplasty technique, and 25 patients were treated with VSP, cutting guides, and a customized plate. Of the total sample, 40% (17 patients) were treated in the context of orthognathic surgery, while 60% of the patients underwent genioplasty for strictly aesthetic reasons.

Only 14% were men (6 patients). The mean age of the patients in the "conventional surgery" group was 28.89 ± 2.26 years; the mean age of the "guided surgery" group was 31.44 ± 1.76 years.

To simplify the study, patients were divided into subgroups: advancement (19 patients), retrusion (13 patients), and rotation (11 patients). The advancement, retrusion, or twist motion is shown in Table S1 (customized guided surgery) and Table S2 (conventional surgery).

3.1. Differences between Planned and Achieved Surgical Motion

The differences between planned and achieved surgical motion (in millimeters) by group is shown in Table 1. There were no significant differences in the comparison of the two techniques with respect to chin advancement or retrusion. However, statistical significance was observed in cases of mandibular asymmetry that required chin rotation ($p = 0.011$).

Table 1. Differences between planned and achieved surgical motion.

	Conventional Genioplasty	Guided Genioplasty	*p* Value
Advance (mm.)	0.13 ± 0.05	0.46 ± 0.02	0.125
Retrusion (mm.)	0.18 ± 0.5	0.10 ±0.06	0.216
Midline change (degrees)	2.60 ± 0.51	0.50 ± 0.22	0.011

3.2. Surgical Time and Hospitalization

The operation time ranged from 35 to 107 min. The mean operative time was 60.06 ± 3.74 min in the conventional surgery group and 42.24 ± 1.29 min in the group treated by VSP, CAD-CAM cutting guides, and a customized plate. There was a considerable decrease in surgical time in the cases treated by guided surgery and individual plate ($p < 0.001$) (Figure 2).

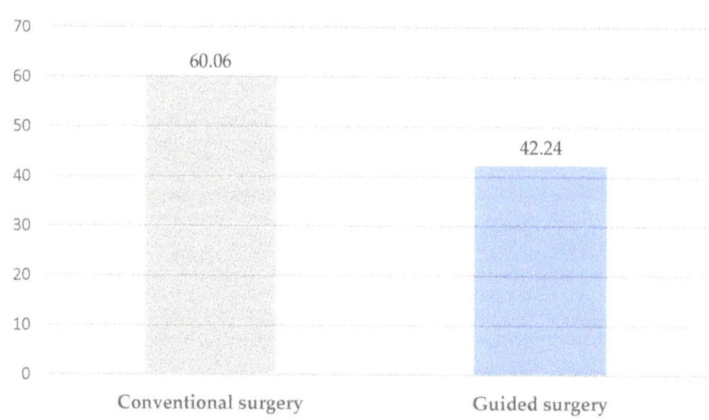

Figure 2. Surgical time (minutes).

The mean hospital stay was 1.4 days, with no differences between groups ($p = 0.196$).

3.3. Aesthetic Outcome: Patient Perception

Eighty-eight percent of the patients (38 cases) considered that they had obtained an "excellent" aesthetic result. Twelve percent (5 cases) evaluated their result as "good". There was no difference between the group treated with conventional surgery and the group treated with customized guided surgery ($p = 0.22$). There was also no statistical difference by subgroup (Table 2).

Table 2. Aesthetic results: patient perception.

	Excellent	Good	Poor
Conventional genioplasty	15	3	0
Guided genioplasty	23	2	0

4. Discussion

The development and refinement of techniques and methods due to technological advances have allowed surgical procedures to be performed with less morbidity, more accurately, and more safely. The use of computer-assisted surgery and navigation technology in head and neck surgery was described at the end of the 20th century by A. Wagner. In recent years, "precision medicine" has been integrated into daily hospital medical practice, allowing the development of specific and customized materials for each case. In this context, maxillofacial surgery as a discipline has benefited from this technological development: virtual surgical planning and the design and manufacture of customized CAD-CAM material have contributed, in recent years, to simplifying and improving the precision of surgeries. Together, all this makes it possible to virtually plan the limits of an osteotomy or a resection, to know the dimensions of a potential defect, to determine the precise location of osteotomies in bone flaps, etc. Cutting guides manufactured using CAD-CAM technology help the surgeon faithfully reproduce the previously planned treatment, improving the precision, accuracy, and reliability of the results in resections and reconstructions of the head and neck area. The combination of VSP and CAD-CAM technology can provide the best possible postoperative results, especially in complex cases without adequate intraoperative anatomical references [10].

There are not many studies describing the use of customized plates and cutting guides in the context of genioplasty; however, there has been an increase in interest in this area in recent years that will make the technique, still susceptible to improvement, be enhanced in the near future. The growing interest and progressive application of virtual surgical planning and the use of customized titanium mini-plates manufactured using CAD-CAM technology have developed in recent years in orthognatic surgery [11–13].

The systematization of the process described in our patients has allowed us to ensure a better result, to increase the precision and safety of the surgery, and to reduce operating room time. This leads to avoid potential peri- and postoperative complications.

Adequate design of the cutting guide is crucial to obtaining a good result. Although it is important to correctly delimit the placement of the osteotomy, it is equally important to take into account the ergonomics and adaptation of the guide to the patient's jaw so as not to collaterally damage important anatomical structures [14]. In our experience and taking into account the idiosyncrasies of each patient as well as the surgeon's preferences, we have designed two types of polyamide cutting guide. One type consists of a two-piece system with intermediate connections and adaptations to the mandibular basal that allow its introduction through a relatively small surgical wound. The other type also has an extension with adjustments to the incisal edge of the teeth of the lower arch to increase stability (Figure 3). In addition, in the design of the guide, it is of vital importance to distribute the holes for fixation to the bone in positions that do not compromise the aesthetic result or damage the mentonian nerves or the floor of the mouth due to excessive length. Attention should also be paid to the length of the titanium screws that will be used to fix the custom osteosynthesis plate. In general, the mandibular bone has a high density, and the bone volume at the mental level is large. However, if the anatomy of each case is not taken into account, it is possible to place screws that are longer than the bone width and cause injury to soft structures, with a potential risk of bleeding, especially the floor of the mouth and the mental area [15,16].

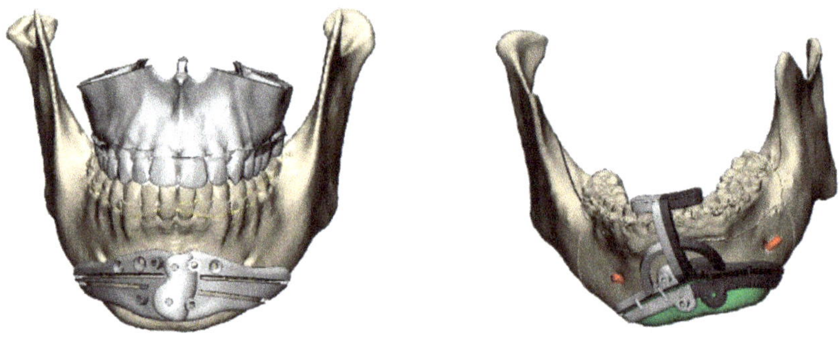

(**a**) (**b**)

Figure 3. Customized guides (Avinent Implant System S.L.U, Santpedor, Barcelona, Spain): (**a**) polyamide customized cutting guide with mandibular adjustment; (**b**) polyamide customized cutting guide with mandibular and teeth adjustment.

The use of polyamide as a material for the manufacture of the customized cutting guides also provides a small modulus of elasticity that enhances the positioning of the instrument at the surgical site and its subsequent adaptation [17,18]. This also makes it possible to maintain a small approach and an earlier recovery of the surgical wound.

We believe there are many advantages to using customized cutting guides when performing mandibular osteotomy. In the conventional technique, the design of the osteotomy is performed "free-hand" according to the surgeon's preference and previous experience; however, the cutting guide ensures an osteotomy path that always avoids the mentonian nerves and the dental apices since they have been previously analyzed in 3D. In addition, it ensures the symmetry of the osteotomy and the precision of the midline positioning. Therefore, the centering of the mentonian bone fragment will also be better positioned [19].

Of course, in cases of asymmetric, complex chins, the placement of the fragment will be much simpler using customized material for the patient according to a previous VSP and will generate less doubt among the surgical team about the final result. This considerably reduces surgical time, as we have demonstrated, and by avoiding excessive manipulation of the soft tissues in cases of disagreement with a conventional procedure, postoperative edema and the sequelae derived from it (pain, swelling, patient discomfort, etc.) are reduced [20]. In our series of cases, there were no statistically significant differences in the cases of chin advancement or retrusion. In this regard, we consider that this may be due to the fact that the movement achieved is equally precise with a previously calibrated chin advancement or retrusion plate. In fact, although it has no clinical relevance, these results may induce the thought that surgery has no benefit in some cases. We believe that the results in simple advancements and retrusions may be slightly inferior in terms of radiologic measurement and comparison—not clinical—than the results obtained in the guided procedures because the latter ones had higher complexity. However, significant differences were found in cases of asymmetry requiring chin rotation, which confirms that planning is especially useful for cases in which the movement is not only in the sagittal plane but in all three dimensions of space.

Undoubtedly, developing genioplasty surgery with cutting guides and customized titanium plates decreases miscalculations and complications with respect to the traditional technique. In the latter case the osteotomy is designed and executed freehand and the fragment is positioned according to the approximate measurement made during the procedure, without having a complete visualization of the structure, which can lead to asymmetric and/or unexpected results, often unacceptable for the patient and the surgeon [21,22].

Complications of genioplasty due to damage to the mentonian nerve or tooth apices are described in the scientific literature with a variation of 3% to 12% [14,23,24]. Although we consider that these are not frequent complications and that, with wide experience, they can be avoided, the safety and precision provided by VSP and the use of this technology during surgical manipulation are unequaled.

In our series, no differences were found with respect to complications, which fortunately were few, although we consider that the safety that the use of customized cutting guides brings to the procedure results in a clear reduction of potential morbidity for the patient. The only relevant complication was a case of mild submental hematoma that was solved conservatively in the conventional surgery group. There were no complications in the group treated with VSP and cutting guides.

In this sense, the aesthetic results obtained are equal to or better than those of the conventional technique and are always more predictable [7,14]. The reduction in surgical time and tissue manipulation resulted in a better and shorter recovery for the patients, although this was a subjective finding on the part of both the patients and the medical team. In any case, the patients' perception of having undergone a more pleasant postoperative period with less swelling than they had expected made their postoperative management as well as their reincorporation into daily life easier.

Related to the use of customized cutting guides, we can affirm that they allow us to design more complex osteotomy paths and to "take better advantage" of the patient's mandibular bone, being able to design more posterior cutting paths that provide more volume and thus avoid the "hourglass" deformity typical of some cases with poor planning [21,24,25].

In addition, in cases of chin advancement and retrusion, the posterior wedges, which are sometimes produced by the movement of the cut area of the bone, are included in the design of the cutting guide, making it possible to achieve a more natural mandibular ridge with a higher-quality aesthetic result. At this point, we consider it important to explain to each patient the steps of their surgical treatment and the normal postoperative findings. In many patients with excellent functional and aesthetic results, there is a complaint of a bony step in the bilateral basal area of the osteotomy. Planned surgery and the use of customized cutting guides allow, in most cases, the design of more posterior osteotomies with a less pronounced gradient toward the mandibular basal that will produce more discrete gaps. However, we insist on informing patients of this possible palpable transition prior to surgery.

In cases of chin asymmetry and also those of mandibular profile, the design of customized cutting guides allows the mandibular contour to be modified with great precision and safety; this would not be possible without the guide since the mandibular basal cannot be visualized during the procedure.

On the other hand, the use of customized titanium plates brings advantages. It reduces the surgical time because, as mentioned above, the placement of the mentonian bone fragment is faster and more precise, and, above all, it will have a positioning in the three dimensions of the space previously defined. In addition, the passive adaptation to the bone surface of the chin and jaw allows for smoother osteosynthesis without potential changes of the designed chin position due to forceful movements to achieve a tighter fit of the titanium screws, thus accidentally bending the titanium mini-plates previously molded on the 3D model or on the patient's bone [10,18].

In our series of cases, a considerable reduction in surgical time has been demonstrated, with the advantages that this entails for the patient. There was no difference in hospitalization time between one case and another. We relate this result to the fact that with both techniques, it is a less aggressive procedure. In addition, many patients who were admitted to the hospital for 1 or 2 days did so for personal reasons and not strictly medical reasons.

The use of VSP, CAD-CAM technology, and customized material allows us to achieve an adequate aesthetic result of the mandibular contour in cases in which the traditional technique produces an unsatisfactory or unpredictable result [21]. It is important to emphasize the high aesthetic demand presented by patients who wish to undergo this procedure in a stand-alone fashion and for aesthetic reasons only.

Despite the great advantages of using this technology, some disadvantages and limitations should also be clarified. First, more time is required for the design of the VSP and the additive manufacturing of the customized models, guides, and plates. We agree with other authors that the whole process can be solved within 48 h [14,26,27]. However, we believe the surgical time saved compensates for the planning effort. This waiting time until virtual surgical planning and obtaining custom cutting guides and titanium plates can be an inconvenience in other contexts. We must consider that this technology applied to the field of genioplasty can be extended to other surgeries in the head and neck area. In interventions that need to be carried out as early as possible (emergencies, oncology patients with potential complex reconstructions of the facial skeleton, accidents in the context of the postoperative period of a surgery that has previously required customized material, etc.), there is the possibility of waiting for the design of the material or, on the contrary, it may be more appropriate to carry out a conventional treatment.

It should be taken into account that the design will not allow intraoperative modifications in case of any error, so that a failure in the planning or an error in the production of the material will mean the need to change the entire preoperative plan. The customized plate must also fit perfectly passively, since it will not allow intraoperative modifications. In these cases, it will be necessary to use one or more conventional osteosynthesis plates [14,28,29].

Although there is an additional cost with the use of this technique (400–1000 euros, according to the authors), there is a savings in anesthetic support in cases performed under local anesthesia and sedation [26,30,31]. In cases performed under general anesthesia, the savings in surgical time will not compensate for the economic expense, but there is a benefit in terms of patient safety and results.

We should mention the limitations of this study. Firstly, this is a study with a small number of cases, so the scope of the results obtained is small. On the other hand, the constant refinement and improvement of the methods means that in each case, details are incorporated into the design of the cutting guides and/or the customized titanium plates that may surpass the previous ones. Although the results obtained are highly satisfactory at the present time, it is expected that a gradual improvement will allow, in a few years, the definition of a standard protocol for guided genioplasty surgery.

Currently, we consider this genioplasty technique superior to the conventional one, so the cases included in this work that were treated by conventional technique are prior to the rest.

5. Conclusions

The multistage application of VSP with CAD-CAM polyamide cutting guides, STL models, and patient-specific titanium plates increases precision in genioplasty surgery, especially in cases of chin asymmetry, reducing operating time and possible complications. The main advantages of this technology are the visualization and preoperative study of the anatomy of each patient, the osteotomy with precise and well-defined limits, the simplification of the surgical technique, the preoperative visualization of the limitations of the case and prevention of potential complications, the reduction of surgical time, and the obtaining of more predictable results. On the other hand, the main disadvantages of virtual surgical planning are increased costs and surgical delays involved in surgical planning and obtaining the different models and guides. Overall, the decrease in patient morbidity and complications and the overall improvement in outcomes could offset the technological costs. Further studies with larger series of patients are needed, as well as improved techniques to standardize the guided surgery protocol to provide better outcomes.

Supplementary Materials: The following supporting information can be downloaded at: https://www.mdpi.com/article/10.3390/jpm13121702/s1. Table S1: Patients treated by customized guided surgery; Table S2: Patients treated by conventional surgery.

Author Contributions: Conceptualization, R.A.-C.H.; methodology, J.A.G.; formal analysis, J.Z.L.; Funding acquisition, M.C.P.; resources, A.L.D. and G.D.M.; data curation, N.N.A., C.S.G.-A., J.A.G., I.N.C., A.L.D. and G.D.M.; writing—original draft preparation, R.A.-C.H. and J.L.S.C.; writing—review and editing, C.N.C.; supervision, R.A.-C.H., C.N.C. and M.C.P. All authors have read and agreed to the published version of the manuscript.

Funding: This research was supported by Avinent Implant System S.L.U, Santpedor, Barcelona, Spain. The company has contributed to the publication of this article. The materials used in the cases presented were designed and manufactured by the company but there has been no funding for the execution of the study.

Institutional Review Board Statement: The study was conducted in accordance with the Declaration of Helsinki, and approved by the Institutional Review Board of Hospital Ruber Juan Bravo, Madrid, Spain (protocol code mxilorjb 1/2024).

Informed Consent Statement: Informed consent was obtained from all subjects involved in the study.

Data Availability Statement: The data presented in this study are available on request from the corresponding author. The data are not publicly available due to data protections regulations.

Conflicts of Interest: The authors declare no conflict of interest.

References

1. Ferretti, C.; Reyneke, J.P. Genioplasty. *Atlas Oral Maxillofac. Surg. Clin. N. Am.* **2016**, *24*, 79–85. [CrossRef] [PubMed]
2. Hofer, O. Operation der Prognathie und Mikrogenie. *Dtsch Zahn Mund Kieferheilkd* **1942**, *9*, 121–132.
3. Gillies, H.; Millard, D.R. *The Principles and Art of Plastic Surgery*; Butterworth: Oxford, UK, 1957.
4. Trauner, R.; Obwegeser, H. The surgical correction of mandibular prognathism and retrognathia with consideration of genioplasty. I. Surgical procedures to correct mandibular prognathism and reshaping of the chin. *Oral Surg. Oral Med. Oral Pathol.* **1957**, *10*, 677–689. [CrossRef] [PubMed]
5. San Miguel Moragas, J.; Oth, O.; Büttner, M.; Mommaerts, M.Y. A systematic review on soft-to-hard tissue ratios in orthognathic surgery part II: Chin procedures. *J. Cranio-Maxillofac. Surg.* **2015**, *43*, 1530–1540. [CrossRef] [PubMed]
6. Antúnez-Conde, R.; Navarro Cuéllar, C.; Salmerón Escobar, J.I.; Díez-Montiel, A.; Navarro Cuéllar, I.; Dell'Aversana Orabona, G.; Del Castillo Pardo de Vera, J.L.; Navarro Vila, C.; Cebrián Carretero, J.L. Intraosseous Venous Malformation of the Zygomatic Bone: Comparison between Virtual Surgical Planning and Standard Surgery with Review of the Literature. *J. Clin. Med.* **2021**, *10*, 4565. [CrossRef] [PubMed]
7. Li, B.; Shen, S.G.; Yu, H.; Li, J.; Xia, J.J.; Wang, X. A new design of CAD/CAM surgical template system for two-piece narrowing genioplasty. *Int. J. Oral Maxillofac. Surg.* **2016**, *45*, 560. [CrossRef] [PubMed]
8. Scolozzi, P. Computer-aided design and computer-aided modeling (CAD/CAM) generated surgical splints, cutting guides and custom-made implants: Which indications in orthognathic surgery? *Rev. Stomatol. Chir. Maxillo-Faciale Chir. Orale* **2015**, *116*, 343. [CrossRef] [PubMed]
9. Shen, P.; Zhao, J.; Fan, L.; Qiu, H.; Xu, W.; Wang, Y.; Zhang, S.; Kim, Y.J. Accuracy evaluation of computer-designed surgical guide template in oral implantology. *J. Cranio-Maxillofac. Surg.* **2015**, *43*, 2189–2194. [CrossRef] [PubMed]
10. Antúnez-Conde, R.; Salmerón, J.I.; Díez-Montiel, A.; Agea, M.; Gascón, D.; Sada, Á.; Navarro Cuéllar, I.; Tousidonis, M.; Ochandiano, S.; Arenas, G.; et al. Mandibular Reconstruction with Fibula Flap and Dental Implants through Virtual Surgical Planning and Three Different Techniques: Double-Barrel Flap, Implant Dynamic Navigation and CAD/CAM Mesh with Iliac Crest Graft. *Front. Oncol.* **2021**, *11*, 719712. [CrossRef]
11. Flügge, T.V.; Nelson, K.; Schmelzeisen, R.; Metzger, M.C. Three-dimensional plot- ting and printing of an implant drilling guide: Simplifying guided implant surgery. *J. Oral Maxillofac. Surg.* **2013**, *71*, 1340–1346. [CrossRef]
12. Kang, S.H.; Lee, J.W.; Lim, S.H.; Kim, Y.H.; Kim, M.K. Validation of mandibular genioplasty using a stereolithographic surgical guide: In vitro comparison with a manual measurement method based on preoperative surgical simulation. *J. Oral Maxillofac. Surg.* **2014**, *72*, 2032–2042. [CrossRef] [PubMed]
13. Olszewski, R.; Tranduy, K.; Reychler, H. Innovative procedure for computer-assisted genioplasty: Three-dimensional cephalometry, rapid-prototyping model and surgical splint. *Int. J. Oral Maxillofac. Surg.* **2010**, *39*, 721–724. [CrossRef]
14. Arcas, A.; Vendrell, G.; Cuesta, F.; Bermejo, L. Mentoplasty with Customized Guides and Plates Using 3D Technology: A More Precise and Safer Technique. *Plast. Reconstr. Surg. Glob. Open* **2019**, *7*, e2349. [CrossRef] [PubMed]
15. Abadi, M.; Pour, O.B. Genioplasty. *Facial Plast. Surg.* **2015**, *31*, 513–522. [PubMed]
16. Keyhan, S.O.; Jahangirnia, A.; Fallahi, H.R.; Navabazam, A.; Ghanean, S. Three-dimensional printer-assisted reduction genioplasty; surgical guide fabrication. *Ann. Maxillofac. Surg.* **2016**, *6*, 278–280. [PubMed]

17. Berridge, N.; Heliotis, M. New technique to improve lower facial contour using a three-dimensional, custom-made, positional stent. *Br. J. Oral Maxillofac. Surg.* **2016**, *54*, 1044–1104. [CrossRef] [PubMed]
18. Yamauchi, K.; Yamaguchi, Y.; Katoh, H.; Takahashi, T. Tooth-bone CAD/CAM surgical guide for genioplasty. *Br. J. Oral Maxillofac. Surg.* **2016**, *54*, 1134–1135. [CrossRef]
19. Aston, S.J.; Smith, D.M. Taking it on the chin: Recognizing and accounting for lower face asymmetry in chin augmentation and genioplasty. *Plast. Reconstr. Surg.* **2015**, *135*, 1591–1595. [CrossRef]
20. Liebregts, J.; Baan, F.; van Lierop, P.; de Koning, M.; Bergé, S.; Maal, T.; Xi, T. One-year postoperative skeletal stability of 3D planned bimaxillary osteotomies: Maxilla-first versus mandible-first surgery. *Sci. Rep.* **2019**, *9*, 3000. [CrossRef]
21. White, J.B.; Dufresne, C.R. Management and avoidance of complications in chin augmentation. *Aesthet. Surg. J.* **2011**, *31*, 634–642. [CrossRef] [PubMed]
22. Khan, M.; Sattar, N.; Erkin, M. Postoperative Complications in Genioplasty and Their Association with Age, Gender, and Type of Genioplasty. *Int. J. Dent.* **2021**, *2021*, 8134680. [CrossRef] [PubMed]
23. Guyot, L. Orthognathic surgery: Surgical failures and complications. *L'Orthodontie Française* **2016**, *87*, 107–109. [CrossRef] [PubMed]
24. Bargi, H.H.A.I.; Suleiman Alshehri, S.A. Massive submentalhematoma, a rare complication after osseous genioplasty. Literature Review and Case Report. *J. Dent. Health Oral Disord. Ther.* **2016**, *5*, 00151. [CrossRef]
25. Bertossi, D.; Albanese, M.; Nocini, R.; Mortellaro, C.; Kumar, N.; Nocini, P.F. Osteotomy in Genioplasty by Piezosurgery. *J. Craniofacial Surg.* **2021**, *32*, e317–e321. [CrossRef]
26. Oth, O.; Mestrallet, P.; Glineur, R. Clinical Study on the Minimally Invasive-Guided Genioplasty Using Piezosurgery and 3D Printed Surgical Guide. *Ann. Maxillofac. Surg.* **2020**, *10*, 91–95. [CrossRef]
27. Lim, S.H.; Kim, M.K.; Kang, S.H. Genioplasty using a simple CAD/CAM (computer-aided design and computer-aided manufacturing) surgical guide. *Maxillofac. Plast. Reconstr. Surg.* **2015**, *37*, 44. [CrossRef]
28. Navarro Cuéllar, C.; Tousidonis Rial, M.; Antúnez-Conde, R.; Ochandiano Caicoya, S.; Navarro Cuéllar, I.; Arenas de Frutos, G.; Sada Urmeneta, Á.; García-Hidalgo Alonso, M.I.; Navarro Vila, C.; Salmerón Escobar, J.I. Virtual Surgical Planning, Stereolitographic Models and CAD/CAM Titanium Mesh for Three-Dimensional Reconstruction of Fibula Flap with Iliac Crest Graft and Dental Implants. *J. Clin. Med.* **2021**, *10*, 1922. [CrossRef]
29. Fleury, C.M.; Sayyed, A.A.; Baker, S.B. Custom Plates in Orthognathic Surgery: A Single Surgeon's Experience and Learning Curve. *J. Craniofacial Surg.* **2022**, *33*, 1976–1981. [CrossRef] [PubMed]
30. Van Sickels, J.E.; Tiner, B.D. Cost of a genioplasty under deep intravenous sedation in a private office versus general anesthesia in an outpatient surgical center. *J. Oral Maxillofac. Surg.* **1992**, *50*, 687–690. [CrossRef]
31. Kumar, P.; Priya, K.; Kirti, S.; Johar, S.; Singh, V. Dexmedetomidine Supported Office Based Genioplasty: A Pilot Study. *J. Maxillofac. Oral Surg.* **2015**, *14*, 750–753. [CrossRef]

Journal of
*Personalized
Medicine*

MDPI

Article

Assessment of Surgical Accuracy in Maxillomandibular Advancement Surgery for Obstructive Sleep Apnea: A Preliminary Analysis

Jean-Pierre T. F. Ho [1,2,3,*], Ning Zhou [1], Tom C. T. van Riet [1,2], Ruud Schreurs [1], Alfred G. Becking [1,2] and Jan de Lange [1,2]

1 Department of Oral and Maxillofacial Surgery, Amsterdam UMC, University of Amsterdam, Meibergdreef 9, 1105 AZ Amsterdam, The Netherlands; n.zhou@amsterdamumc.nl (N.Z.); t.c.vanriet@amsterdamumc.nl (T.C.T.v.R.); r.schreurs@amsterdamumc.nl (R.S.); j.delange@amsterdamumc.nl (J.d.L.)
2 Academic Centre for Dentistry of Amsterdam (ACTA), University of Amsterdam and Vrije Universiteit Amsterdam, 1081 LA Amsterdam, The Netherlands
3 Department of Oral and Maxillofacial Surgery, Northwest Clinics, Wilhelminalaan 12, 1815 JD Alkmaar, The Netherlands
* Correspondence: j.p.ho@amsterdamumc.nl

Abstract: This retrospective study aimed to: (1) investigate the surgical accuracy of maxillomandibular advancement (MMA) in obstructive sleep apnea (OSA) patients, with a specific focus on maxillary and mandibular advancement and counter-clockwise rotation and (2) investigate the correlation between the amount of achieved advancement and the reduction in the relative apnea hypopnea index (AHI). Sixteen patients, for whom a three-dimensional virtual surgical plan was generated preoperatively and a computed tomography scan (CT) or cone-beam computer tomography (CBCT) was acquired postoperatively, were included. The postoperative CT or CBCT was compared to the virtual surgical plan, and differences in the mandibular and maxillary advancement and counter-clockwise rotation were assessed. Maxillary and mandibular advancement (median 3.1 mm, $p = 0.002$ and 2.3 mm, $p = 0.03$, respectively) and counter-clockwise rotation (median 3.7°, $p = 0.006$ and 4.7°, $p = 0.001$, respectively) were notably less than intended. A significant correlation was found between the planned maxillary advancement and the difference between the planned and actual maxillary advancement ($p = 0.048$; adjusted $R^2 = 0.1979$) and also between the planned counter-clockwise rotation and the difference between the planned and actual counter-clockwise rotation for the mandible ($p = 0.012$; adjusted $R^2 = 0.3261$). Neither the maxilla-first nor the mandible-first surgical sequence proved to be superior in terms of the ability to achieve the intended movements ($p > 0.45$). Despite a significant reduction ($p = 0.001$) in the apnea hypopnea index (AHI) from a median of 62.6 events/h to 19.4 events/h following MMA, no relationship was found between the extent of maxillary or mandibular advancement and AHI improvement in this small cohort ($p = 0.389$ and $p = 0.387$, respectively). This study underlines the necessity for surgeons and future research projects to be aware of surgical inaccuracies in MMA procedures for OSA patients. Additionally, further research is required to investigate if sufficient advancement is an important factor associated with MMA treatment outcome.

Keywords: obstructive sleep apnea; surgery; orthognathic surgical procedures; osteotomy; accuracy

1. Introduction

Obstructive sleep apnea (OSA) is a sleep-related breathing disorder characterized by repeated partial or complete obstruction of the upper airway, leading to hypopneas or apneas [1]. Patients frequently suffer from excessive daytime sleepiness, fatigue, tiredness, snoring, gasping, and morning headaches [2]. Risk factors for OSA mainly include older age, male sex, obesity, smoking, alcohol use, family history of OSA, and craniofacial and upper airway morphology [3–5].

For decades, the preferred first-line treatment option for moderate-to-severe OSA has been nonsurgical 'continuous positive airway pressure' (CPAP) [6–8]. Another common non-invasive option for OSA treatment is the use of a mandibular advancement device (MAD) [9]. A disadvantage of CPAP and MAD is suboptimal long-term adherence. Surgical therapy provides a solution for OSA patients who have difficulties accepting lifelong treatment with CPAP or MAD. In an American Academy of Sleep Medicine clinical practice guideline, it is recommended that clinicians discuss and/or refer adult OSA patients with a body mass index (BMI) < 40 kg/m^2 who are intolerant or unaccepting of positive airway pressure (PAP) to a sleep surgeon for an alternative treatment options, as part of a patient-oriented solution [10].

Maxillomandibular advancement surgery (MMA) has proven to be the most effective surgical treatment for OSA—aside from tracheostomy—with a success rate of approximately 85% [8,11–13]. The surgical procedure consists of a combination of a Le Fort I osteotomy for the maxilla and a bilateral sagittal split osteotomy (BSSO) for the mandible. The maxilla and mandible are both significantly advanced and rotated counter-clockwise to enlarge the upper airway's volume and reduce upper airway soft tissue collapsibility [13–15]. Virtual surgical planning (VSP) is used for preoperative simulation of the MMA, and 3D-printed surgical splints are generated from the VSP to transfer the plan to the surgical setting [16]. Since large maxillomandibular complex advancement and counter-clockwise rotation contribute to a decrease in the apnea hypopnea index (AHI) and therefore treatment success, achieving these planned movements accurately during surgery is essential [12,17]. Previous research has shown that the planned surgical movements are often not accurately achieved in standard orthognathic surgery, especially in cases with larger movements [18]. Given the extensive movements involved in MMA, it is reasonable to expect that the planned movements in MMA might be even less accurately achieved compared to standard orthognathic surgery. Surprisingly, no prior studies have investigated the extent to which planned—specifically sagittal—movements are accurately achieved in MMA procedures.

The primary aim of this study was to investigate the extent to which planned advancement and counter-clockwise rotation, the two most relevant movements for surgical success in MMA for OSA surgery, are accurately achieved. The secondary aim of this study was to investigate the correlation between realized maxillary and mandibular advancement and relative AHI reduction.

2. Materials and Methods

2.1. Study Participants

Patients treated for OSA with MMA in the Department of Oral and Maxillofacial Surgery of the Amsterdam University Medical Centers (UMC) between November 2017 and March 2020 were considered for inclusion in this study. The inclusion criteria were: (1) adults aged 18 years or older; (2) diagnosed with OSA through polysomnography (PSG); (3) CPAP therapy failure or intolerance; (4) PSG conducted at least 3 months postoperatively; (5) preoperative three-dimensional (3D) virtual surgical planning of MMA; and (6) availability of a spiral computed tomography (CT) or cone-beam computer tomography (CBCT) scan after surgery. Exclusion criteria were: (1) patients undergoing other additional procedures during MMA (e.g., multi-piece Le Fort osteotomy, temporomandibular joint (TMJ) reconstruction); (2) previous Le Fort I osteotomy or BSSO; (3) cleft palate or syndromic patients; and (4) insufficient image quality for postoperative analysis. The study design was a retrospective cohort study.

This study was conducted and performed in accordance with the Declaration of Helsinki guidelines for human research. Patients were sent a letter to inform them that their medical records, polysomnography results, and radiological images were anonymously going to be used for study purposes. The option was provided to opt out of inclusion in the study. Included patients' medical records were reviewed and data were collected. Preoperative (baseline) patient characteristics included gender, age, and body mass index (BMI).

The Medical Ethics Committee of the Amsterdam UMC decided that this study was waived for the Medical Research Human Subjects Act (W22_042 # 22.07).

2.2. Imaging Protocol

CT (Somatom Force, Siemens Medical Solutions, Erlangen, Germany) or CBCT (Planmeca Promax, Planmeca OY, Helsinki, Finland) scans were acquired 1 to 6 weeks preoperatively using a standardized protocol (120 kV, 300 mAs, field of view (FOV) 240 mm, pitch 0.55, slice thickness 1.0 mm, image matrix 512 × 512, window W1600/L400, hard-tissue kernel (Hr64)) or CBCT scan (84–96 kV, 100 mAs, FOV 230 mm × 170 mm (diameter × height), slice thickness 0.4 mm, image matrix 575 × 575, window/level 2500/596, pixel size 0.4 mm). Scanned patients were instructed to remain still, relax, and place the bite in a retruded contact position.

Baseline two-dimensional skeletal patterns and relationships were obtained on lateral cephalometric radiographs between 1 and 6 weeks preoperatively. Steiner radiographic cephalometric analyses were performed in Viewbox (version 4; dHAL Software, Kifissia, Greece).

2.3. Virtual Surgical Planning

Preoperative CT or CBCT data were exported in digital imaging and communications in medicine (DICOM) format and imported into the Maxilim software (Medicim NV, Mechelen, Belgium) (until April 2017) or IPS CaseDesigner (KLS Martin, Tuttlingen, Germany) (from May 2017 onwards). A 3D virtual patient model was reconstructed and aligned with the patient's natural head position (NHP) based on clinical assessment and standardized patient photos [19]. The maxilla and mandible were virtually osteotomized according to a Le Fort I osteotomy and BSSO, respectively (Figure 1). Based on the planned maxillary and mandibular position, intermediate and final splints were designed and 3D-printed for either maxilla-first or mandible-first treatment sequence based on the surgeon's preference.

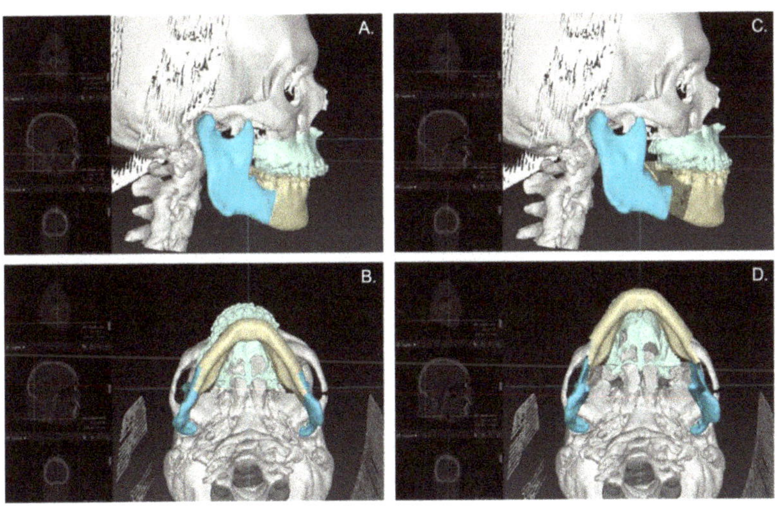

Figure 1. An example of a virtual plan of an MMA case. Lateral (**A**) and caudal (**B**) view of the preoperative 3D virtual hard-tissue skull model of the patient in IPS (KLS Martin, Tuttlingen, Germany). Lateral (**C**) and caudal (**D**) view of the postoperative 3D virtual hard-tissue skull model, where the maxilla and mandible are virtually osteotomized according to a Le Fort I osteotomy and BSSO. The maxilla and mandible are advanced and counter-clockwise pitched.

2.4. Surgical Technique

2.4.1. Le Fort I Osteotomy

A gingivobuccal incision was made, apical, from the first molar on the right to the first molar on the left. Subperiosteal dissection and elevation of the oral soft tissue and nasal mucosa were performed. A Le Fort I osteotomy was performed using a reciprocating saw from the pterygoid processes towards the piriform rims. A glabella reference marker was placed. Down-fracturing and mobilization of the maxilla was performed with a bone hook and Rowe's forceps. A surgical splint was used to position the maxilla in the intended planned position after the removal of interferences. Temporary maxillomandibular fixation was performed using power chains or steel wire ligatures. Rigid fixation was applied with an array of titanium miniplates and monocortical screws. Wound closure followed with absorbable sutures.

2.4.2. Bilateral Sagittal Split Osteotomy (BSSO)

A mucosal incision was made with subperiosteal dissection and elevation of the oral soft tissue along the anterior border on one side of the ramus and continued inferiorly, along the external oblique ridge. A horizontal, oblique, and vertical osteotomy was placed with either a burr or reciprocating saw according to the Hunsuck modification of the Obwegeser and Dal Pont BSSO technique [20]. The bone segments were separated with osteotomes and a bone spreader. The same procedure was applied on the contralateral side. A surgical splint was used to position the mandible in the planned position, and rigid fixation was applied with an array of titanium miniplates and monocortical or bicortical screws after putting the maxillomandibular complex into temporary maxillomandibular fixation with power chains or steel wire ligatures. Wound closure followed with absorbable sutures.

In the maxilla-first surgical protocol, the Le Fort I osteotomy was performed before the BSSO, and in the mandible-first protocol, the BSSO was performed before the Le Fort I osteotomy. Antibiotics (Augmentin, GlaxoSmithKline BV, Zeist, The Netherlands) were administered at the start of the procedure and continued for 7 days postoperatively. All patients were monitored for at least one night in the intensive care or medium care unit [21].

2.5. Outcome Evaluation

In order to evaluate the accuracy of the achieved postoperative result, the preoperative and postoperative DICOM data were imported into 3D MedX (3D Lab Radboudumc, Nijmegen, the Netherlands) to assess the surgical result with the OrthoGnathicAnalyser workflow [18,22]. This is a validated evaluation tool, which is able to calculate the transformation between the planned and achieved maxilla and mandible and express the deviation in clinically relevant parameters: (1) front–back translation (posteroanterior axis); (2) right–left translation (lateromedial axis); (3) up–down translation (superoinferior axis); (4) roll; (5) pitch; and (6) yaw (Figure 2). The main goal in MMA surgery is to adequately advance the maxilla and mandible and rotate them counter-clockwise in order to enlarge the upper airway. It is therefore essential to achieve the planned advancement and counter-clockwise rotation; thus, these were the parameters that were investigated in this study.

Patients received a full-night level 1 (in lab) or 2 (at home) PSG prior to MMA surgery and at least 3 months after surgery (Somnoscreen; SOMNOmedics GmbH, Randersacker, Germany). To assess sleep stages, EEG (F3, F4, C3, C4, M1, M2, O1, O2), EOG, and submental EMG were used. Nasal airflow was measured with a cannula/pressure transducer. Oronasal thermal flow determined airflow and mouth breathing. Arterial oxyhemoglobin was monitored via pulse oximetry. Thoracoabdominal excursions were measured qualitatively with respiratory belts. A position sensor determined body position, and limb movements were detected with tibial EMG. Cardiac events were scored via ECG, and snoring was recorded with a snore sensor. A clinical neurophysiologist specialized in scoring sleep studies interpreted and scored the sleep studies based on the updated 2007 criteria from the American Academy of Sleep Medicine [23]. Included PSG parameters consisted of the preoperative and postoperative apnea hypopnea index (AHI), 3% oxygen desaturation index (ODI), and lowest oxygen saturation (LSAT). According to Sher's criteria, surgical response was defined as "at least 50% AHI reduction following MMA and a postoperative AHI < 20" [24].

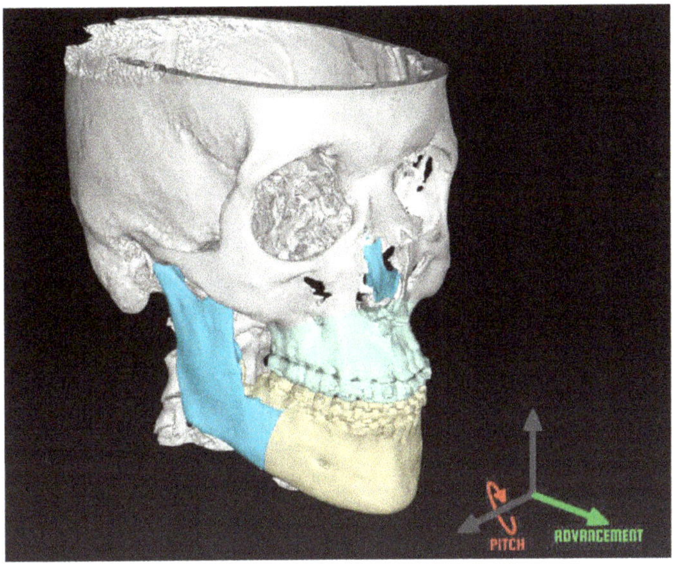

Figure 2. Maxillomandibular complex positioning frame. The back-to-front (advancement) translation is shown in green and pitch rotation is shown in red around the reference axes.

2.6. Sample Size

Due to the nature of retrospective design, the sample size was not estimated prior to the study. A post hoc power analysis was performed for the primary outcome variables (i.e., observed differences between planned and achieved movements) using G*Power (Version 3.1.9.6, Heinrich-Heine-Universität Düsseldorf, Düsseldorf, Germany).

2.7. Statistical Analysis

Statistical analysis was performed using SPSS (version 29.0; IBM Corp., Armonk, NY, USA) and R (R Development Core Team, Vienna, Austria). Descriptive statistics were calculated for all demographic and outcome variables. Mean, standard deviation, median, interquartile range (IQR), and/or range were used to report the continuous variables, and frequency and percentage were used for summarizing categorical variables. Normality was tested using the Shapiro–Wilk test. To compare the paired continuous values, the paired-samples t-test (for data with a normal distribution) or Wilcoxon's signed-rank test (for non-normal data) were used. To compare continuous values between the maxilla-first and mandible-first surgical sequence group, the independent-samples t-test was used when data were normally distributed, and the Mann–Whitney U test was used when data were not normally distributed. Linear regression analysis was performed to investigate the association between the planned movement and the difference between the planned and achieved movement. Adjusted R-squared (R^2) value was used to quantify the proportion of the variance that could be explained by the planned movement in the linear regression model. The relative AHI improvement was calculated, and a Pearson correlation analysis was used to investigate its relationship with the amount of maxillary and mandibular advancement. For all analyses, a p-value < 0.05 was considered statistically significant.

3. Results

3.1. Study Participants

In total, 27 patients underwent MMA for OSA in the Department of Oral and Maxillofacial Surgery, Amsterdam UMC, between November 2017 and March 2020. One patient opted out of the study, and ten patients were excluded due to the fact that the 3D-imaging protocol was not followed correctly, which was mostly due to the absence of a CT or CBCT scan after surgery ($n = 7$). Therefore, 16 patients were included in this study; 10 were male and 6 were female. The mean age was 53 ± 9 years (range 36–69 years) (Table 1). Among the included sixteen patients, all patients (100%) had treatment failure or intolerance to CPAP, twelve patients (75%) had treatment failure or intolerance to MAD, and seven patients (44%) had other type(s) of upper airway surgery prior to MMA.

Table 1. Baseline characteristics of the study population.

Total Population ($n = 16$)		Mean ± SD	Range
Male (n (%))	10 (62.5)		
Age (years)		52.9 ± 9.3	36–69
BMI (kg/m^2)		27.1 ± 3.9	18.0–32.4
∠SNA (degrees)		80.40 ± 3.9	69.6–88.1
∠SNB (degrees)		73.9 ± 7.4	52.0–83.8
∠ANB (degrees)		6.1 ± 5.0	−0.1–17.7
∠OP-SN (degrees)		20.8 ± 12.0	5.0–59.9
∠MP-SN (degrees)		42.5 ± 16.3	13.6–90.5

Gender is presented as number of patients and percentage. Age, BMI, ∠SNA, ∠SNB, ∠ANB, ∠OP-SN, and ∠MP-SN are presented in years, kg/m^2, and degrees. ∠ANB, angle between the A/nasion plane and the nasion/B plane; BMI, body mass index; cm, centimeters; kg/m^2, kilograms per square meter; ∠MP-SN, angle between the mandibular plane and the sella/nasion plane; ∠OP-SN, angle between the occlusal plane and the sella/nasion plane; SD, standard deviation; ∠SNA, angle between the sella/nasion plane and the nasion/A plane; ∠SNB, angle between the sella/nasion plane and the nasion/B plane. p-value < 0.05 was considered statistically significant.

3.2. Planned vs. Realized Movements

The median planned advancement of the maxilla was 9.5 mm (range 6.0–12.0 mm), and the median planned advancement for the mandible was 11.2 mm (range 4.9–18.4 mm). The planned median counter-clockwise rotation for the maxilla and mandible were 6.2° (range 0.0–10.2°) and 7.8° (range 1.2–25.4°), respectively. For both the maxilla and mandible, the achieved advancement and counter-clockwise rotation were significantly smaller than the planned advancement and rotation ($p < 0.05$) (Table 2). The study revealed that a larger advancement corresponded to a larger difference between the planned and realized advancement for both the maxilla and mandible. Notably, this difference was only found to be statistically significant for the maxilla ($p = 0.048$; adjusted $R^2 = 0.20$) and not for the mandible ($p = 0.06$; adjusted $R^2 = 0.18$) (Figure 3). A larger counter-clockwise rotation was associated with a significantly greater difference between the planned and realized counter-clockwise rotation for the mandible ($p = 0.012$; adjusted $R^2 = 0.33$) but not for the maxilla ($p = 0.9$; adjusted $R^2 = 0.07$) (Figure 4).

3.3. Maxilla-First Surgical Sequence vs. Mandible-First Treatment Sequence

In the comparative analysis between the maxilla-first surgical sequence and the mandible-first treatment sequence, Table 3 serves to demonstrate their collective inability to achieve the intended movements accurately. In the analysis, the discrepancies between the planned and achieved movements between the maxilla-first and mandible-first surgical sequences were all not statistically significantly ($p > 0.45$).

Table 2. Comparison between planned and achieved advancement (B-F translation) and counter-clockwise rotation (anticlockwise pitch) for maxilla and mandible.

		Planned			Achieved			Difference			p-Value
		Median	**IQR**	**Range**	**Median**	**IQR**	**Range**	**Median**	**IQR**	**Range**	
Counter-clockwise rotation (degrees)	Maxilla	6.2	3.9–7.7	0.0–10.2	2.6	0.7–5.6	4.8–13.7	3.7	1.7–6.2	−6.1–7.9	0.006
	Mandible	7.8	6.3–11.0	1.2–25.4	4.5	2.6–6.2	−5.7–14.9	4.7	1.2–8.2	−0.8–10.5	0.001
Advancement (mm)	Maxilla	9.5	7.9–11.9	6.0–12.0	6.7	5.7–8.2	1.4–9.5	3.1	2.1–4.3	0.6–12.0	0.002
	Mandible	11.2	8.7–13.3	4.9–18.4	8.7	7.9–9.9	1.7–16.9	2.3	0.3–4.6	−3.1–6.4	0.03

Translations are presented in mm. Rotations are presented in degrees. B-F translation, translation from back to front; mm, millimeters; IQR, interquartile range = quartile 3—quartile 1. p-value < 0.05 was considered statistically significant.

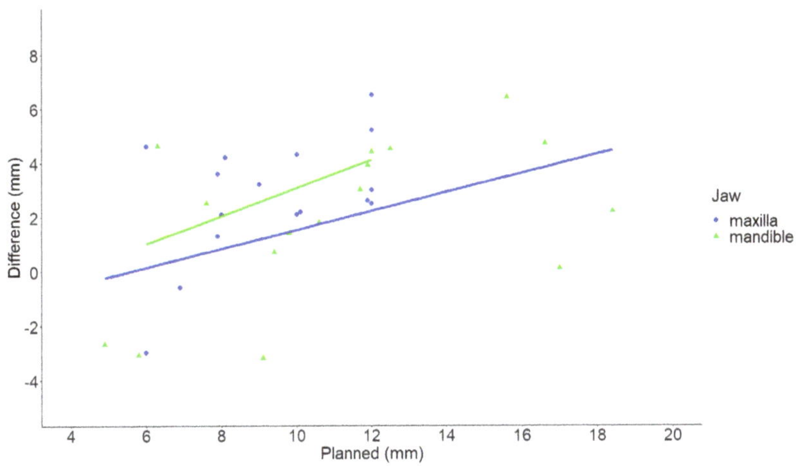

Figure 3. Scatter plot illustrating the relationship between the planned advancement and the difference between planned and realized advancement. The X-axis illustrates the planned advancement in mm. The Y-axis illustrates the difference between planned and realized advancement in mm. Each green triangle depicts an individual maxilla, and each blue dot depicts an individual mandible. The green and blue lines illustrate the linear regression of the maxilla and mandible data, respectively. Mm, millimeters. p-value < 0.05 was considered statistically significant.

Table 3. Comparison of discrepancies between planned and achieved sagittal movements in maxilla-first vs. mandible-first surgical sequences.

		Maxilla-First (n = 7)			Mandible-First (n = 9)			p-Value
		Median	**IQR**	**Range**	**Median**	**IQR**	**Range**	
Counter-clockwise rotation (degrees)	Maxilla	4.3	2.5–6.5	0.3–7.8	2.8	1.2–6.8	0.6–7.9	0.71
	Mandible	4.5	3.3–8.7	0.8–9.2	4.8	0.7–7.3	0.0–10.5	0.50
Advancement (mm)	Maxilla	3.1	2.1–4.3	2.1–5.1	2.6	1.7–4.1	0.6–6.5	0.66
	Mandible	1.8	1.4–4.6	0.1–4.6	3.1	2.4–4.3	0.7–6.4	0.45

Rotations are presented in degrees. Translations are presented in mm. B-F translation, translation from back to front; mm, millimeters; IQR, interquartile range = quartile 3—quartile 1. p-value < 0.05 was considered statistically significant.

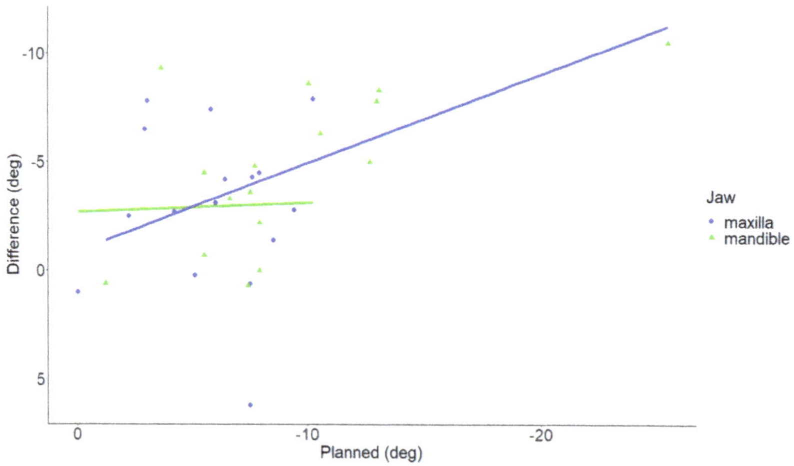

Figure 4. Scatter plot illustrating the relationship between the planned counter-clockwise rotation and the difference between planned and realized counter-clockwise rotation. The X-axis illustrates the planned pitch in deg. The Y-axis illustrates the difference between planned and realized counter-clockwise rotation in deg. Each green triangle depicts an individual maxilla, and each blue dot depicts an individual mandible. The green and blue lines illustrate the linear regression of the maxilla and mandible data, respectively. Deg, degree. p-value < 0.05 was considered statistically significant.

3.4. *Amount of Advancement and the Relative AHI Improvement*

The median AHI was significantly reduced from 62.6 (6.4–84.0) events/h to 19.4 (3.9–47.0) events/h ($p = 0.001$). Overall success was achieved in 63% of the cases (Table 4).

Table 4. PSG results before and after MMA for total population.

	Total Population ($n = 16$)				
	Mean	**SD**	**Median**	**IQR**	**Range**
Pre-op AHI (events/h)	49.8	23.8	62.6	43.5–77.7	6.4–84.0
Post-op AHI (events/h)	17.3	12.8	19.4	10.8–29.9	3.9–47.0
Pre-op ODI (events/h)	50.9	25.8	64.7	45.6–75.8	2.2–93.4
Post-op ODI (events/h)	21.0	13.9	19.5	10.5–31.8	3.0–51.1
Pre-op LSAT (%)	74.7	12.0	76	63–80	52–92
Post-op LSAT (%)	82.4	8.8	85	75–87	64–92
Success (%)	10/16 (62.5)				
Cure (%)	3/16 (18.8)				

PSG results are presented as events/hour or percentage. Success and cure are presented as percentage. AHI; apnea hypopnea index; events/h, post-op, after MMA; pre-op, prior to MMA; N, number of patients; LSAT, lowest oxygen saturation; MMA, maxillomandibular advancement; ODI, oxygen desaturation index; PSG, polysomnography; IQR, interquartile range = quartile 3—quartile 1; SD, standard deviation. p-value < 0.05 was considered statistically significant.

No association was found between the amount of realized maxillary and mandibular advancement and the relative AHI improvement ($p = 0.389$ and $p = 0.387$ respectively) (Figure 5).

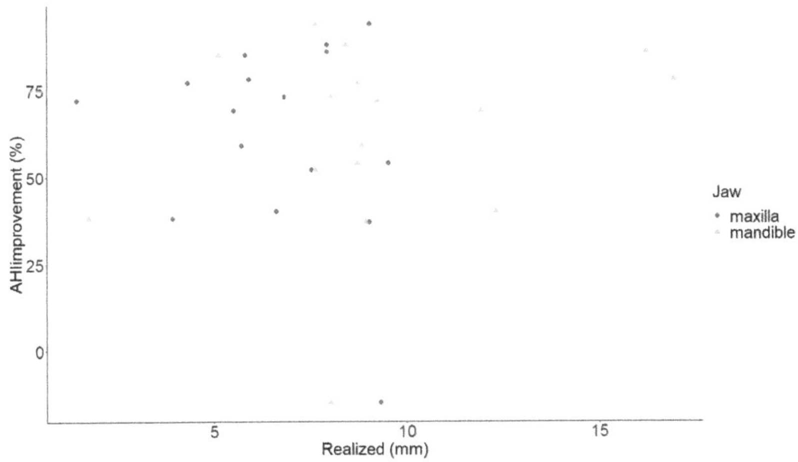

Figure 5. Scatter plot illustrating the relationship between the realized maxillary and mandibular advancement and the percentage of AHI improvement. The X-axis illustrates the realized advancement in mm. The Y-axis illustrates the AHI improvement in %. Each green triangle depicts an individual maxilla, and each blue dot depicts an individual mandible. AHI, apnea hypopnea index; mm, millimeters; %, percentage. *p*-value < 0.05 was considered statistically significant.

4. Discussion

Previous studies have looked into the accuracy of orthognathic surgery [18,22,25,26]. However, as far as the authors are aware of, none have explored the extent to which planned surgical movements are accurately achieved in MMA procedures [17,18]. Therefore, the present study aimed to investigate the extent to which preoperative planned advancements and counter-clockwise rotations were achieved during MMA surgery for OSA patients.

One of the main findings of this preliminary study is the consistent trend of under-achievement of the desired advancements in the MMA cases. This is well in line with findings in traditional orthognathic surgery for the correction of dentofacial discrepancies [22]. Notably, these discrepancies may be attributed to various factors, for example altered seated position of the condyle as a result of different muscular tone and patient positioning intraoperatively [22,27].

In addition to the difference found between the planned and realized advancement, the results also show that the realized counter-clockwise rotation for both the maxilla and mandible were consistently less than planned. Liebregts et al. found a similar difference between the planned and realized counter-clockwise rotation in bimaxillary osteotomies in traditional orthognathic surgery [18]. The possible reasons for this might be positioning errors intraoperatively due to interfering bone segments between the osteotomized maxilla and the pterygoid plates or a non-centric relation of the mandible during temporary maxillomandibular fixation with the use of intraoperative surgical splints [18,22].

Both findings emphasize that although virtual surgical planning and CAD/CAM intraoperative surgical splints are utilized for MMA nowadays, it is still difficult to accurately achieve the planned advancement and counter-clockwise rotation. The relatively large surgical splints that are frequently used in MMA surgery, due to the large planned displacements, might be a significant factor in decreasing surgical accuracy. This might explain the results of this study, which showed that the surgical accuracy was further reduced when the planned advancements and counter-clockwise rotations increased. The paper by Liebregts et al. and Stokbro et al. also alluded to this finding [18,28].

The mandible-first sequence has been proposed as a solution to address issues with centric relation and, consequently, to enhance the predictability of achieving the intended position [29]. However, no significant beneficial effect could be demonstrated in this small sample size. The choice between the maxilla-first and mandible-first surgical sequences is often influenced by surgeon preferences [30,31]. In cases of OSA, concerns about achieving the desired maxillary advancement due to limitations in soft tissue (e.g., through scarring due to previous upper airway surgery) might be present. In our hospital, a strategic approach is often used that is only possible within the maxilla-first sequence. It involves the use of two intermediate splints: one for larger advancement (e.g., 12 mm) and another for a slightly lesser advancement (e.g., 10 mm) as a precautionary 'back-up'.

Multiple studies have reported the association between MMA success and the amount of advancement [12,17], but others have reported no association between the amount of planned advancement and AHI improvement after MMA [32,33]. A possible explanation for these inconsistent findings could be that the planned advancement instead of the realized advancement has been used, or because there is variation in the use of two-dimensional and three-dimensional imaging methods [17,34,35].

As a secondary objective, this study investigated the correlation between the realized advancement and the relative AHI reduction, but no significant correlation was found. This lack of correlation may be attributed to the low number of patients included and the extensive complexity of OSA, where treatment success or improvement depends on various interacting factors, including demographic characteristics, anatomical hard-tissue and soft-tissue parameters, PSG specifics, and surgical characteristics [35–39]. This finding raises the question of whether or not more accurate achievement of the planned advancement and counter-clockwise rotation is actually necessary through, for example, a splintless surgical workflow [40–43]. This is especially true when looking at the finding that the median AHI was significantly reduced from approximately 63 events/h to 19 events/h despite consistently not achieving the planned displacements. Some cases still showed a significant relative AHI reduction despite a small advancement, as seen in Figure 5.

The amount of advancement and counter-clockwise rotation necessary for surgical success remains unknown. A major advantage of the present study is the fact that a validated workflow and tool, the OrthoGnathicAnalyser, was used in order to measure the discrepancy between the planned and the realized result in three dimensions with the use of CT and CBCT. The argument could be raised that an error distribution between the CT- and CBCT-based registration could have influenced the outcome of this study. However, based on the validated findings of Eggers et al. this can be considered as negligible [44]. Although the OrthoGnathicAnalyser tool is able to accurately measure all translational and rotational movements, the main focus in this study was on the advancement and the counter-clockwise rotation of the maxilla and the mandible, as these are essential factors contributing to the relief of patients' OSA [14,45–48]. However, caution is warranted in interpreting the results because of the study limitations (small population, potential biases in retrospective design, and low inclusion rate). In the present study, the powers of the primary outcomes (i.e., maxillary advancement, mandibular advancement, maxillary counter-clockwise rotation, and mandibular counter-clockwise rotation) were 1, 0.7, 0.8, and 1, respectively. This indicated that except for mandibular advancement, all other primary outcome variables had sufficient power in the statistical analyses. It is recommended that future studies—preferably prospective studies in large cohorts—should be undertaken to verify the current findings, especially since the literature on the topic is scarce. Additional future research should further investigate which factors in MMA surgery contribute most to surgical success and to optimize surgical planning for individual patients.

5. Conclusions

This study emphasizes the importance of acknowledging the presence of surgical inaccuracies in MMA procedures for patients with OSA and underscores the need for heightened awareness among surgeons and future research endeavors. Furthermore, our findings propose that the extent of maxillomandibular complex advancement may not hold paramount significance in determining the outcome of MMA treatment. Therefore, further investigations and refinements in surgical techniques are imperative to optimize the efficacy of MMA procedures.

Author Contributions: Conceptualization, J.-P.T.F.H., T.C.T.v.R. and R.S.; methodology, J.-P.T.F.H., T.C.T.v.R. and R.S.; formal analysis, J.-P.T.F.H., T.C.T.v.R., N.Z. and R.S.; investigation, J.-P.T.F.H., N.Z., T.C.T.v.R. and R.S.; data curation, J.-P.T.F.H., N.Z. and R.S.; writing—original draft preparation, J.-P.T.F.H., N.Z., T.C.T.v.R., R.S., A.G.B. and J.d.L.; writing—review and editing, J.-P.T.F.H., N.Z., T.C.T.v.R., R.S., A.G.B. and J.d.L. All authors have read and agreed to the published version of the manuscript.

Funding: This research received no external funding.

Institutional Review Board Statement: This study was deemed not to be subject to the Medical Research Human Subjects Act by the Medical Ethics Committee of the Amsterdam University Medical Centers (UMC), location Academic Medical Center (AMC) (reference number W22_042 # 22.07). Therefore, formal approval was waived.

Informed Consent Statement: Informed consent was obtained from all subjects involved in the study.

Data Availability Statement: The data presented in this study are available on request from the corresponding author.

Acknowledgments: The authors thank C. Klop and J. Sabelis for their assistance with the analysis of the cases and N. Su for his help and guidance with the statistics analysis used in this study.

Conflicts of Interest: The authors declare no conflict of interest.

References

1. Malhotra, A.; White, D.P. Obstructive sleep apnoea. *Lancet* **2002**, *360*, 237–245. [CrossRef] [PubMed]
2. Gottlieb, D.J.; Punjabi, N.M. Diagnosis and Management of Obstructive Sleep Apnea: A Review. *JAMA* **2020**, *323*, 1380–1400. [CrossRef] [PubMed]
3. Young, T.; Skatrud, J.; Peppard, P.E. Risk factors for obstructive sleep apnea in adults. *JAMA* **2004**, *291*, 2013–2016. [CrossRef] [PubMed]
4. Dastan, F.; Ghaffari, H.; Shishvan, H.H.; Zareiyan, M.; Akhlaghian, M.; Shahab, S. Correlation between the upper airway volume and the hyoid bone position, palatal depth, nasal septum deviation, and concha bullosa in different types of malocclusion: A retrospective cone-beam computed tomography study. *Dent. Med. Probl.* **2021**, *58*, 509–514. [CrossRef]
5. Tofangchiha, M.; Esfehani, M.; Eftetahi, L.; Mirzadeh, M.; Reda, R.; Testarelli, L. Comparison of the pharyngeal airway in snoring and non-snoring patients based on the lateral cephalometric study: A case-control study. *Dent. Med. Probl.* **2023**, *60*, 121–126. [CrossRef]
6. Sullivan, C.E.; Berthon-Jones, M.; Issa, F.G.; Eves, L. Reversal of Obstructive Sleep Apnoea by Continuous Positive Airway Pressure Applied Through the Nares. *Lancet* **1981**, *317*, 862–865. [CrossRef]
7. Patil, S.P.; Ayappa, I.A.; Caples, S.M.; John Kimoff, R.; Patel, S.R.; Harrod, C.G. Treatment of adult obstructive sleep apnea with positive airway pressure: An American academy of sleep medicine systematic review, meta-analysis, and GRADE assessment. *J. Clin. Sleep. Med.* **2019**, *15*, 301–334. [CrossRef]
8. Epstein, L.J.; Kristo, D.; Strollo, P.J.; Friedman, N.; Schwab, R.J.; Weaver, E.M.; Weinstein, M.D. Clinical guideline for the evaluation, management and long-term care of obstructive sleep apnea in adults. *J. Clin. Sleep. Med.* **2009**, *5*, 263–276. [CrossRef]
9. Marklund, M.; Verbraecken, J.; Randerath, W. Non-CPAP therapies in obstructive sleep apnoea: Mandibular advancement device therapy. *Eur. Respir. J.* **2012**, *39*, 1241–1247. [CrossRef]
10. Kent, D.; Stanley, J.; Aurora, R.N.; Levine, C.; Gottlieb, D.J.; Spann, M.D.; Torre, C.A.; Green, K.; Harrod, C.G. Referral of adults with obstructive sleep apnea for surgical consultation: An American Academy of Sleep Medicine clinical practice guideline. *J. Clin. Sleep. Med.* **2021**, *17*, 2499–2505. [CrossRef]
11. Zhou, N.; Ho, J.-P.T.F.; Huang, Z.; Spijker, R.; De Vries, N.; Aarab, G.; Lobbezoo, F.; Ravesloot, M.J.L.; de Lange, J. Maxillomandibular advancement versus multilevel surgery for treatment of obstructive sleep apnea: A systematic review and meta-analysis. *Sleep. Med. Rev.* **2021**, *57*, 101471. [CrossRef] [PubMed]
12. Holty, J.E.C.; Guilleminault, C. Maxillomandibular advancement for the treatment of obstructive sleep apnea: A systematic review and meta-analysis. *Sleep. Med. Rev.* **2010**, *14*, 287–297. [CrossRef] [PubMed]
13. Zaghi, S.; Holty, J.E.C.; Certal, V.; Abdullatif, J.; Guilleminault, C.; Powell, N.B.; Camacho, M. Maxillomandibular advancement for treatment of obstructive sleep apnea a meta-analysis. *JAMA Otolaryngol. Head. Neck Surg.* **2016**, *142*, 58–66. [CrossRef]
14. Liu, S.Y.C.; Awad, M.; Riley, R.W. Maxillomandibular Advancement: Contemporary Approach at Stanford. *Atlas Oral. Maxillofac. Surg. Clin. North. Am.* **2019**, *27*, 29–36. [CrossRef] [PubMed]
15. Li, K.K. Surgical management of obstructive sleep apnea. *Clin. Chest Med.* **2003**, *24*, 365–370. [CrossRef] [PubMed]

16. Randerath, W.; de Lange, J.; Hedner, J.; Ho, J.-P.T.F.; Marklund, M.; Schiza, S.; Steier, J.; Verbraecken, J. Current and Novel Treatment Options for OSA. *ERJ Open Res.* **2022**, *8*, 00126–02022. [CrossRef]
17. Rubio-Bueno, P.; Landete, P.; Ardanza, B.; Vázquez, L.; Soriano, J.B.; Wix, R.; Capote, A.; Zamora, E.; Ancochea, J.; Naval-Gías, L. Maxillomandibular advancement as the initial treatment of obstructive sleep apnoea: Is the mandibular occlusal plane the key? *Int. J. Oral Maxillofac. Surg.* **2017**, *46*, 1363–1371. [CrossRef]
18. Liebregts, J.; Baan, F.; De Koning, M.; Ongkosuwito, E.; Bergé, S.; Maal, T.; Xi, T. Achievability of 3D planned bimaxillary osteotomies: Maxilla-first versus mandible-first surgery. *Sci. Rep.* **2017**, *7*, 9314. [CrossRef]
19. Cassi, D.; De Biase, C.; Tonni, I.; Gandolfini, M.; Di Blasio, A.; Piancino, M.G. Natural position of the head: Review of two-dimensional and three-dimensional methods of recording. *Br. J. Oral Maxillofac. Surg.* **2016**, *54*, 233–240. [CrossRef]
20. Böckmann, R.; Meyns, J.; Dik, E.; Kessler, P. The modifications of the sagittal ramus split osteotomy: A literature review. *Plast. Reconstr. Surgery Glob. Open* **2014**, *2*, e271. [CrossRef]
21. Ravesloot, M.J.L.; de Raaff, C.A.L.; van de Beek, M.J.; Benoist, L.B.L.; Beyers, J.; Corso, R.M.; Edenharter, G.; Haan, C.D.; Azad, J.H.; Ho, J.-P.T.F.; et al. Perioperative Care of Patients with Obstructive Sleep Apnea Undergoing Upper Airway Surgery. *JAMA Otolaryngol. Neck Surg.* **2019**, *145*, 751–760. [CrossRef]
22. Baan, F.; Liebregts, J.; Xi, T.; Schreurs, R.; De Koning, M.; Bergé, S.; Maal, T. A new 3D tool for assessing the accuracy of bimaxillary surgery: The OrthoGnathicanAlyser. *PLoS ONE* **2016**, *11*, e0149625. [CrossRef] [PubMed]
23. Berry, R.B.; Budhiraja, R.; Gottlieb, D.J.; Gozal, D.; Iber, C.; Kapur, V.K.; Marcus, C.L.; Mehra, R.; Parthasarathy, S.; Tangredi, M.M.; et al. Rules for scoring respiratory events in sleep: Update of the 2007 AASM Manual for the Scoring of Sleep and Associated Events. Deliberations of the Sleep Apnea Definitions Task Force of the American Academy of Sleep Medicine. *J. Clin. Sleep Med.* **2012**, *8*, 597–619. [CrossRef] [PubMed]
24. Sher, A.E.; Schechtman, K.B.; Piccirillo, J.F. The efficacy of surgical modifications of the upper airway in adults with obstructive sleep apnea syndrome. *Sleep* **1996**, *19*, 156–177. [CrossRef] [PubMed]
25. Hsu, S.S.-P.; Gateno, J.; Bell, R.B.; Hirsch, D.L.; Markiewicz, M.R.; Teichgraeber, J.F.; Zhou, X.; Xia, J.J. Accuracy of a computer-aided surgical simulation protocol for orthognathic surgery: A prospective multicenter study. *J. Oral Maxillofac. Surg.* **2013**, *71*, 128–142. [CrossRef] [PubMed]
26. Liebregts, J.; Baan, F.; van Lierop, P.; de Koning, M.; Bergé, S.; Maal, T.; Xi, T. One-year postoperative skeletal stability of 3D planned bimaxillary osteotomies: Maxilla-first versus mandible-first surgery. *Sci. Rep.* **2019**, *9*, 3000. [CrossRef]
27. Lee, C.-Y.; Jang, C.-S.; Kim, J.-W.; Kim, J.-Y.; Yang, B.-E. Condylar repositioning using centric relation bite in bimaxillary surgery. *Korean J. Orthod.* **2013**, *43*, 74–82. [CrossRef]
28. Stokbro, K.; Liebregts, J.; Baan, F.; Bell, R.B.; Maal, T.; Thygesen, T.; Xi, T. Does Mandible-First Sequencing Increase Maxillary Surgical Accuracy in Bimaxillary Procedures? *J. Oral Maxillofac. Surg.* **2019**, *77*, 1882–1893. [CrossRef]
29. Pampín Martínez, M.M.; Gutiérrez Venturini, A.; de Cevallos, J.; Blanco, M.B.; Niño, I.A.; Sánchez, A.M.; Vera, J.L.d.C.P.d.; Carretero, J.L.C. Evaluation of the Predictability and Accuracy of Orthognathic Surgery in the Era of Virtual Surgical Planning. *Appl. Sci.* **2022**, *12*, 4305. [CrossRef]
30. Perez, D.; Ellis, E., 3rd. Sequencing bimaxillary surgery: Mandible first. *J. Oral Maxillofac. Surg.* **2011**, *69*, 2217–2224. [CrossRef]
31. Turvey, T. Sequencing of two-jaw surgery: The case for operating on the maxilla first. *J. Oral Maxillofac. Surg.* **2011**, *69*, 2225. [CrossRef] [PubMed]
32. Smatt, Y.; Ferri, J. Retrospective study of 18 patients treated by maxillomandibular advancement with adjunctive procedures for obstructive sleep apnea syndrome. *J. Craniofac. Surg.* **2005**, *16*, 770–777. [CrossRef] [PubMed]
33. De Ruiter, M.H.T.; Apperloo, R.C.; Milstein, D.M.J.; de Lange, J. Assessment of obstructive sleep apnoea treatment success or failure after maxillomandibular advancement. *Int. J. Oral Maxillofac. Surg.* **2017**, *46*, 1357–1362. [CrossRef] [PubMed]
34. Lye, K.W.; Waite, P.D.; Meara, D.; Wang, D. Quality of life evaluation of maxillomandibular advancement surgery for treatment of obstructive sleep apnea. *J. Oral Maxillofac. Surg.* **2008**, *66*, 968–972. [CrossRef]
35. Zhou, N.; Ho, J.-P.T.F.; Visscher, W.P.; Su, N.; Lobbezoo, F.; de Lange, J. Maxillomandibular advancement for obstructive sleep apnea: A retrospective prognostic factor study for surgical response. *Sleep. Breath. October* **2022**, *27*, 1567–1576. [CrossRef]
36. Chang, J.L.; Alt, J.A.; Alzoubaidi, M.; Ashbrook, L. International Consensus Statement on Obstructive Sleep Apnea. *Int. Forum Allergy Rhinol.* **2023**, *13*, 1061–1482. [CrossRef]
37. Ho, J.-P.T.F.; Zhou, N.; de Lange, J. Obstructive Sleep Apnea Resolution in Hypopnea-Predominant versus Apnea-Predominant Patients after Maxillomandibular Advancement. *J. Clin. Med.* **2023**, *12*, 311. [CrossRef]
38. Ho, J.T.F.; Zhou, N.; Verbraecken, J.; Vries, N.; de Lange, J. Central and mixed sleep apnea related to patients treated with maxillomandibular advancement for obstructive sleep apnea : A retrospective cohort study. *J. Cranio-Maxillofacial Surg.* **2022**, *50*, 537–542. [CrossRef]
39. Vonk, P.E.; Rotteveel, P.J.; Ravesloot, M.J.L.; Ho, J.P.T.F.; de Lange, J.; de Vries, N. The influence of position dependency on surgical success in patients with obstructive sleep apnea undergoing maxillomandibular advancement. *J. Clin. Sleep. Med.* **2020**, *16*, 73–80. [CrossRef]
40. Suojanen, J.; Leikola, J.; Stoor, P. The use of patient-specific implants in orthognathic surgery: A series of 30 mandible sagittal split osteotomy patients. *J. Cranio-Maxillofacial Surg.* **2017**, *45*, 990–994. [CrossRef]
41. Li, B.; Shen, S.; Jiang, W.; Li, J.; Jiang, T.; Xia, J.; Wang, X. A new approach of splint-less orthognathic surgery using a personalized orthognathic surgical guide system: A preliminary study. *Int. J. Oral Maxillofac. Surg.* **2017**, *46*, 1298–1305. [CrossRef] [PubMed]

42. Kraeima, J.; Jansma, J.; Schepers, R.H. Splintless surgery: Does patient-specific CAD-CAM osteosynthesis improve accuracy of Le Fort I osteotomy? *Br. J. Oral Maxillofac. Surg.* **2016**, *54*, 1085–1089. [CrossRef] [PubMed]
43. Ho, J.P.T.F.; Schreurs, R.; Baan, F.; De Lange, J. Splintless orthognathic surgery in edentulous patients—A pilot. *Int. J. Oral Maxillofac. Surg.* **2019**, *49*, 587–594. [CrossRef]
44. Eggers, G.; Senoo, H.; Kane, G.; Mühling, J. The accuracy of image guided surgery based on cone beam computer tomography image data. *Oral Surg. Oral Med. Oral Pathol. Oral Radiol. Endod.* **2009**, *107*, e41–e48. [CrossRef] [PubMed]
45. Liu, S.Y.C.; Awad, M.; Riley, R.; Capasso, R. The Role of the Revised Stanford Protocol in Today's Precision Medicine. *Sleep Med. Clin.* **2019**, *14*, 99–107. [CrossRef] [PubMed]
46. Knudsen, T.B.; Laulund, A.S.; Ingerslev, J.; Homøe, P.; Pinholt, E.M. Improved apnea-hypopnea index and lowest oxygen saturation after maxillomandibular advancement with or without counterclockwise rotation in patients with obstructive sleep apnea: A meta-analysis. *J. Oral Maxillofac. Surg.* **2015**, *73*, 719–726. [CrossRef]
47. Jeong, W.S.; Kim, Y.C.; Chung, Y.S.; Lee, C.Y.; Choi, J.W. Change in Posterior Pharyngeal Space after Counterclockwise Rotational Orthognathic Surgery for Class II Dentofacial Deformity Diagnosed with Obstructive Sleep Apnea Based on Cephalometric Analysis. *J. Craniofac. Surg.* **2017**, *28*, e488–e491. [CrossRef]
48. Wei, S.; Zhang, Y.; Guo, X.; Yu, W.; Wang, M.; Yao, K.; Sun, H.; Zhang, H.; Lu, X. Counterclockwise maxillomandibular advancement: A choice for Chinese patients with severe obstructive sleep apnea. *Sleep Breath.* **2017**, *21*, 853–860. [CrossRef]

Journal of *Personalized Medicine*

MDPI

Article

Safety and Aesthetics of Autologous Dermis-Fat Graft after Parotidectomy: A Multidisciplinary Retrospective Study

Ciro Emiliano Boschetti [1], Rita Vitagliano [1,*], Nicola Cornacchini [1], Mario Santagata [1], Valentina Caliendo [2], Maria Paola Belfiore [2], Giuseppe Colella [1], Gianpaolo Tartaro [1] and Salvatore Cappabianca [2]

1 Oral and Maxillofacial Surgery Unit, Multidisciplinary Department of Medical-Surgical and Dental Specialties, University of Campania "Luigi Vanvitelli", 80131 Naples, Italy; ciroemiliano.boschetti@unicampania.it (C.E.B.); nicola.cornacchini@studenti.unicampania.it (N.C.); mario.santagata@unicampania.it (M.S.); giuseppe.colella@unicampania.it (G.C.); gianpaolo.tartaro@unicampania.it (G.T.)

2 Department of Precision Medicine, University of Campania Luigi Vanvitelli, Piazza Luigi Miraglia, 80138 Naples, Italy; valentina.caliendo@unicampania.it (V.C.); mariapaola.belfiore@unicampania.it (M.P.B.); salvatore.cappabianca@unicampania.it (S.C.)

* Correspondence: rita.vitagliano@studenti.unicampania.it; Tel.: +39-3271321309

Abstract: (1) Background: In surgical procedures for maxillofacial tumours, it is challenging to preserve functional and cosmetic properties in the affected patients. The use of fat grafting is considered as a valuable alternative to overcome postoperative aesthetic asymmetry problems. (2) Methods: In this study, we enrolled thirty patients with parotid gland tumours in which a partial or complete parotidectomy was performed with positioning in the parotid bed of autologous dermis-fat grafts. We evaluated the satisfaction rate of the patients and the objective efficacy in solving the deformity by comparing MRI data before and after surgery. (3) Results: Twenty-six patients showed a satisfying cosmetic result with proper facial symmetry between the affected side and the healthy one. Two patients presented mild postsurgical complications such as haematomas, and two patients reported temporary weakness of the facial nerve related to the parotidectomy. (4) Conclusions: Based on the imaging data obtained via MRI before and after surgery, we can assess that the employment of fat grafts in parotidectomy surgical procedures gives good cosmetic results and does not affect the post operative management and follow up of oncologic patients.

Keywords: reconstructive surgery; oncologic head and neck surgery; fat graft; parotidectomy; head and neck MRI

1. Introduction

Parotid gland tumours are considered a medical condition that, most of the time, requires surgical treatment by performing a partial or complete parotidectomy.

This surgical procedure represents a challenge for head and neck surgeons because of the anatomical location of the parotid gland. Some tumours are literally surrounded by a complex network of facial nerves branches, and the main difficulty is the performance of a tumour resection while avoiding nervous lesions and preserving nervous integrity and functionality as much as possible. However, due to the anatomical, aesthetical, and functional complexity of the region, there are important cosmetic implications after the removal of a parotid gland tumour, as the resectioning of parotid tumours has been shown to cause facial depression deformities [1]. As a matter of fact, many parotid tumours could reach massive dimensions, causing not only a concern for the general behaviour of the tumour and its tempestive eradication but also causing a visible facial deformity and asymmetry that would negatively affect patients' social lives [2]. When a parotid gland tumour with relevant dimensions is removed, it leaves a depression in the preauricular and infra-auricular region that could create facial deformities and asymmetry and could potentially create aesthetical discomfort in the patients after surgery [3]. In order to avoid a poor cosmetic result that may severely decrease a patient's quality of life and self-esteem, especially in young patients [4], the evaluation of a quick, safe, satisfactory, and cost-effective reconstructive option could be necessary. Thus, according to a few authors, this reconstructive procedure should be performed during the same operating session immediately after the tumour resection, as implanting grafts in the affected anatomical area could immediately overcome any cosmetic defect; also, a single parotidectomy and a parotidectomy with the harvesting and implanting of a reconstructive graft have similar operation times [1,5,6]. Different types of materials and grafts can be employed for the reconstruction of facial soft tissue defects, such as alloplastic materials (polyethylene, silicone, or polyacrylamide), or grafts, such as superficial temporal fascia flaps, sternocleidomastoid muscle flaps [7], superficial muscular aponeurotic system (SMAS) flaps, and free fat grafts [8,9]. In our study, in all patients, the postresection defect was treated with free autologous dermis-fat grafts.

Our multidisciplinary study aimed to demonstrate, in our experience, how this century-old milestone in craniofacial reconstructive surgery has a complete oncological safety profile during the surgery and for the oncological follow up, and it is also a reliable procedure for surgeons, without the lengthening of surgical times, and has a low rate of complications and a high aesthetical satisfaction rate for the patients.

2. Materials and Methods

In our study, thirty patients with parotid gland tumours were enrolled from February 2019 to May 2022, who received a partial or complete parotidectomy with contemporary reconstruction with autologous en bloc dermal fat grafts. Twenty-two of these patients had a benign lesion, and the remaining eight patients had a malignant tumour. The surgical procedure consisted of a classic Blair incision with the sub-surface dissection of the musculoaponeurotic system, the identification of the tumour and its isolation from the surrounding nerve structures, tumour resection, and en bloc dermal fat grafting. The facial nerve trunk and its branches were found and preserved in each case. In all cases, we preferred to obtain the en bloc dermal fat graft through a linear suprapubic incision with a minimum length of 6 cm, which would be individually shaped according to the size of the defect of each patient, and we carefully closed the surgical access with cosmetic intradermal sutures with no drainage. After the harvesting process of the autologous en bloc dermal fat graft from the suprapubic region (Figure 1), the graft was irrigated with antibiotic-soaked saline and contoured with scissors to fit the anatomical region and cover the defect. A 'monobloc' de-epithelialisation technique was performed, involving the removal of the epidermal layer as a whole with a scalpel, on the en bloc autologous dermal fat graft in all cases (Figure 2a) [10].

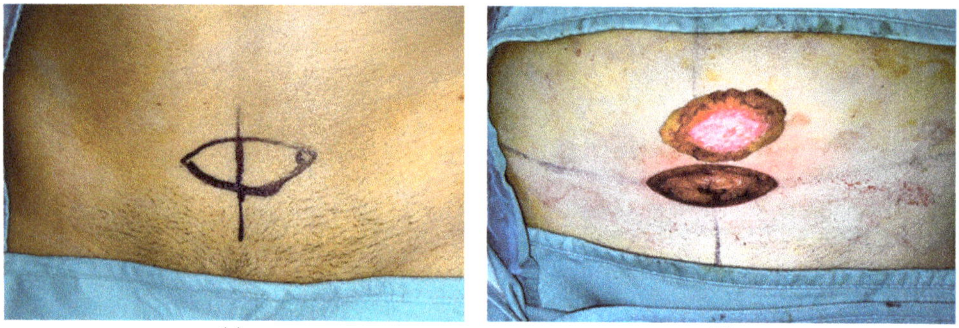

(a) (b)

Figure 1. The en bloc fat graft design and harvesting. (**a**) Patient 1. Surgical design of the en bloc fat graft with a linear sovrapubic incision. (**b**) Patient 2. Surgical harvesting of the en bloc autologous fat graft after de-epithelialisation process.

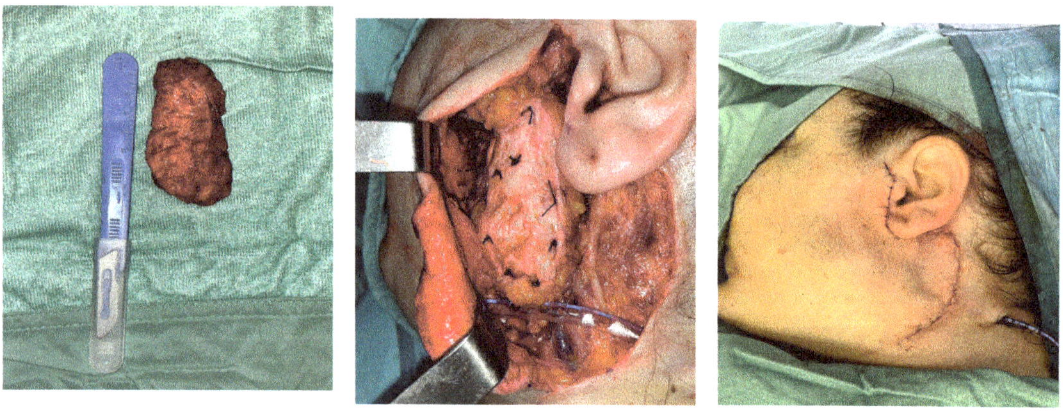

(a) (b) (c)

Figure 2. The en bloc fat graft design and harvesting. (**a**) Patient 1. En bloc fat graft obtained from the sovrapubic region after the de-epithelialisation process. (**b**) Patient 1. Surgical fixation process of the en bloc autologous fat graft to the surgical gap after parotidectomy. (**c**) Patient 1. Closure of the surgical site after the fixation process of the en bloc autologous fat graft and the placement of the drainage.

After the shaping process of the autologous fat graft according to the size of the defect and its positioning in the postparotidectomy surgical gap, we fixated it to the parotid residual bed with absorbable sutures (Figure 2b); the SMAS flap was used as a cover of the dermis-fat graft to give a vascular supply, and then, we placed a drainage in the parotid site for a minimum of 24 h, considering less than 20 mL of serosanguineous fluid an indication for its removal (Figure 2c).

The postoperative management included local cooling application, 3 days of antibiotic therapy, and 20 days of therapy with dietary supplements composed of escin and bromelain supplements (Floganday®, Maya Pharma, Naples, Italy) in order to contain the oedema. Exclusion criteria were patients who had preoperative planning of neck dissection, in order to avoid the risk of an increase in perioperative and postoperative complications, and patients over 80 years of age. The whole procedure for obtaining the en bloc autologous dermis-fat graft was performed simultaneously to the parotidectomy and it did not represent a time-prolongating factor for the whole surgical session. MRI was performed before the surgery, and 60 days, 6 months, and one year after surgery for the oncological follow up, to determine proper facial symmetry and tissue density to achieve a satisfying cosmetic result. No touch-up procedures were performed after surgery. With data obtained with MRI, we were able to perform mirroring by superimposing images before and after surgery and objectively assessing the effective compensation of the defect with dermis-fat grafting, and in the long-term follow up, we approximately evaluated whether there was fat reabsorption.

3. Results

Thirty patients, twenty females and ten males, were enrolled in this study. Their age ranged from 14 to 78 years old. All patients were Caucasian, except one patient, who was of African descent. Twenty-two patients had benign lesions, and eight had malignant lesions (Table 1).

Table 1. Patients' characteristics, including gender, age, parotid first-step surgery (1: partial parotidectomy; 2: superficial parotidectomy; 3: total parotidectomy), and final histologic diagnosis.

Patient	Gender	Age	Extent of Surgery (P.P. [1], S.P. [2], T.P. [3])	Final Histologic Diagnosis
1	F	49	P.P.	Pleomorphic adenoma
2	F	28	P.P.	Pleomorphic adenoma
3	F	14	P.P.	Pleomorphic adenoma
4	F	73	P.P.	Warthin tumour
5	M	54	T.P.	Mucoepidermoid carcinoma
6	M	78	T.P.	Salivary duct carcinoma
7	M	69	T.P.	Metastatic squamous cell carcinoma
8	F	21	T.P.	Acinic cell carcinoma
9	M	51	P.P.	Warthin tumour
10	M	21	P.P.	Pleomorphic adenoma
11	F	64	P.P.	Warthin tumour
12	F	48	P.P.	Warthin tumour
13	F	56	S.P.	Carcinoma ex pleomorphic adenoma
14	F	33	S.P.	Myoepithelioma
15	M	51	T.P.	Salivary duct carcinoma
16	F	37	S.P.	Pleomorphic adenoma (recurrency)
17	M	67	T.P.	Pleomorphic adenoma (recurrency)
18	F	55	T.P.	Pleomorphic adenoma
19	F	59	S.P.	Mucoepidermoid carcinoma (low grade)
20	M	65	P.P.	Solitary Extrapleural Fibrous Tumour
21	F	53	S.P.	Myoepithelioma
22	F	75	S.P.	Myoepithelioma
23	M	63	S.P.	Basal cells adenoma
24	F	37	P.P.	Warthin tumour
25	F	76	S.P.	Myoepithelioma
26	M	45	S.P.	Pleomorphic adenoma
27	F	62	P.P.	Pleomorphic adenoma
28	F	52	P.P.	Warthin tumour
29	F	44	S.P.	Pleomorphic adenoma
30	F	42	S.P.	Acinic cell carcinoma

Tumours were resected without damaging the surrounding facial nerve branches, only in five cases were the ipsilateral facial nerve or its inferior branches (the marginalis mandibulae or the buccalis branches) strictly adherent to the neoplasms and correctly isolated without direct damage to the branches of the facial nerve. In all cases, the en bloc dermis-fat graft was obtained via a suprapubic incision; in three female patients, the incision was performed on a previously existing scar. The hospitalization time for all the patients was three days. The short-term follow up was performed after three days, seven days, ten days, and fourteen days after hospital discharge. The long-term follow up was performed after three, six, and twelve months. Two patients reported, as an early complication, haematoma in the parotidectomy area after the surgery in the first week after surgery; in both cases, this complication was successfully treated with light compressive treatment and escin and bromelain ointment (Floganday®) three times per day for 2 weeks. One patient reported facial nerve weakness related to the surgical procedure used for the removal of the tumour, which was strictly adherent to the network of several facial nerve branches; it involved the mandibular branch and completely resolved over a maximal duration of one month, with the application of Kabat therapy [11] and the use of oral corticosteroid therapy and vitamin "B-complex" supplements [12]. We did not observe complications with the fat graft such as infections, liquefaction, or graft loss due to excessive fat resorption [13,14]. We asked the patients to answer a satisfaction questionnaire with a score ranging from 0 to 5. According to the patients that decided to participate in our questionnaire, twelve patients gave a score of 5/5; four patients gave a score of 4/5; three patients gave a score of 3/5; two patients gave a score of 2/5; one patient gave a score of 1/5. We documented the preoperative and postoperative courses of patients through frontal facial, lateral facial, and semi-lateral facial pictures, and with these pictures, we reported the facial expression before and after surgery to assess nervous integrity (Figure 3).

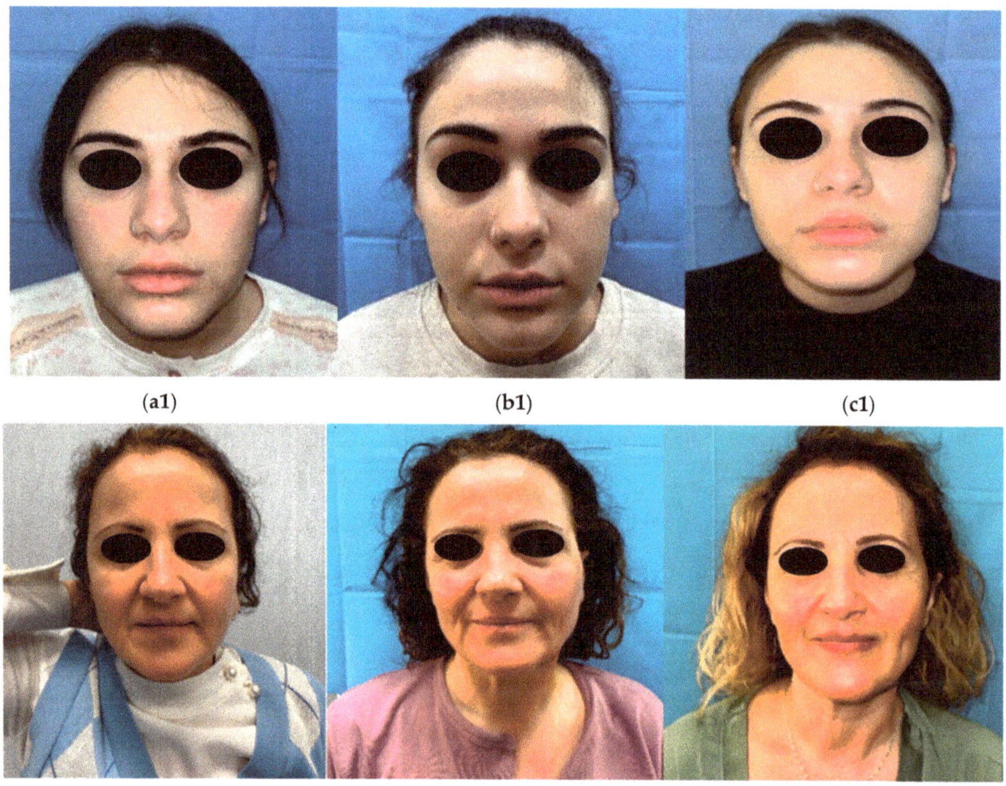

(a1) (b1) (c1)

(a2) (b2) (c2)

Figure 3. Sequence of clinical assessment of facial symmetry before surgery (**a1**,**a2**), 7 days after surgery (**b1**,**b2**), and during 3-month follow-up after surgery (**c1**,**c2**) in patient 1 (**upper** row) and patient 2 (**lower** row).

4. Discussion

The German surgeon Gustav Neuber was the first to describe and use a free fat autografting technique in 1893 [15]. He transplanted adipose tissue from a patient's arm to the orbit to cosmetically improve the sequelae associated with osteomyelitis. Since then, fat grafting has become a progressively employed technique for reconstructive surgery in maxillofacial procedures, like, for example, in case of facial contouring, radiation damage, burn injuries, parotidectomies, or the surgical treatment of MRONJ [16,17]. Fat tissue has a very similar texture and consistency to the parotid tissue [1], representing an ideal substitute in the case of a partial or complete parotidectomy. The donor sites are usually covered body parts such as the abdominal, gluteal, iliac, or sacral region. The final decision about the donor site for an en bloc autologous dermis-fat graft is influenced by the fat volume required, relying on the first-step surgical procedure applied (partial or complete parotidectomy); then, the fat volume of the donor site based on the location of excess adipose tissue is evaluated for each patient case-by-case and is based on both surgeon and patient preferences. In our patients, we always obtained the en bloc autologous dermis-fat graft with a linear incision from the suprapubic lower abdominal region because it is a body part usually easily covered by clothes or underwear, it has easy and fast surgical access, and it also leaves a minimally visible scar with a cosmetic intradermic suture. It is also a saving-time reconstructive option that does not increase the length of surgery. The time taken to harvest and de-epthelially engraft the en bloc autologous dermis fat graft, in our cases, was always about forty-five minutes, and it could be performed simultaneously to the parotidectomy; the autologous en bloc fat graft, as a low-complexity technique, could also easily be a suitable reconstructive alternative for patients with comorbidities and poor systemic conditions [18]. The en bloc autologous dermis-fat graft technique is also very useful to prevent a few postoperative complications of parotidectomy, like Frey's Syndrome or facial haematomas or blood loss [19,20].

We also found that in three patients who underwent an autologous fat graft who had a mild facial nerve injury (HB scale I-II), with the help of our protocol of Kabat therapy [21], they had a faster recovery time for the weakness of the facial nerve, plausibly related to the protective effect of the fat graft on the nerve; according to few authors, this could be correlated to native adipose-derived stem cells present in the transferred tissue, which could potentially act upon regenerating axons, but conclusions are still not completely clear, and studies are still in progress (Figure 3) [22].

Considering the reabsorption rate of fat grafting, we collected more fat with an over-approximation between 20 and 30%. Complications associated with parotidectomy reconstruction with a fat graft are haematoma in the donor site, fat graft necrosis and liquefaction, surgical sutures' dehiscence, cutaneous complications in the donor site such as itching, hypoesthesia, and hypersensitivity [17]. The most unpredictable complication associated with a fat graft is the rate of resorption in the postoperative period [14]. This resorption can potentially range from 0% to 100%, making the whole procedure have unsatisfactory results, because if the reabsorbed fat is excessive, the depression is not compensated for, and aesthetic symmetry not respected. In our study, patients with malignant lesions were involved, because, based on the recommendations of our radio diagnostic team, fat tissue is clearly distinguishable from malignant tumour tissue in MRI [3,5], dispelling the concept that fat grafting should be avoided in patients with malignancies because the reconstruction can mask the tumour identification in postoperative diagnostic imaging. This gave us the "green light" to proceed with fat grafting on patients with malignant tumours.

4.1. The Radiologist's Perspective

4.1.1. MRI Protocol

All patients underwent contrast-enhanced MRI of the face and neck before and after parotidectomy.

MRI examinations were performed on a 1.5 T scanner (SIGNA Voyager, GE Healthcare, Chicago, IL, USA) using a phased-array head and neck coil. The MRI protocol consisted of T1-weighted (T1W) fast spin echo (FSE) (TR/TE: 551.0/9.2 ms), T2-weighted (T2W) fast spin echo (FSE) (TR/TE: 8994.0/83.1 ms), and T2W STIR (TR/TE: 14,878.0/68.6 ms) sequences in the axial plane with 3 mm slice thickness.

DWI was performed with an echoplanar SE sequence (TR/TE, 14,782/66.8 ms; FOV, 22 × 22 cm^2; matrix, 128 × 128; NEX, 2; slice thickness, 3 mm) in the axial plane with two different b-values (0 and 1000 s/mm^2). Finally, fat-saturated isotropic 3D T1w GRE sequences (LAVA) on the axial plane were obtained before and after the intravenous injection of 0.2 mL/kg of Gadoteric Acid (Claricyclic, GE Healthcare, Chicago, IL, USA) at 2.0 mL/s. Multiplanar reconstructions on the coronal and sagittal plane were subsequently performed.

In postoperative studies, the volume of the reconstructed parotid gland was determined through semi-automatic segmentation at the workstation (aycan Worskstation, aycan Medical Systems, Rochester, New York, USA). Finally, a volumetric comparison with the contralateral parotid gland was performed.

4.1.2. MRI Analysis

MR image analysis was performed by two radiologists with >2 years of experience in head and neck radiology.

Fat has an unequivocal appearance on MRI, as it shows high signal intensity on spin echo T1- and T2-weighted images and rather homogeneous signal loss on fat-suppressed sequences, with no contrast enhancement or restricted diffusion. Thanks to these features, dermal fat grafts were easily identified in all the postoperative studies (Figure 4).

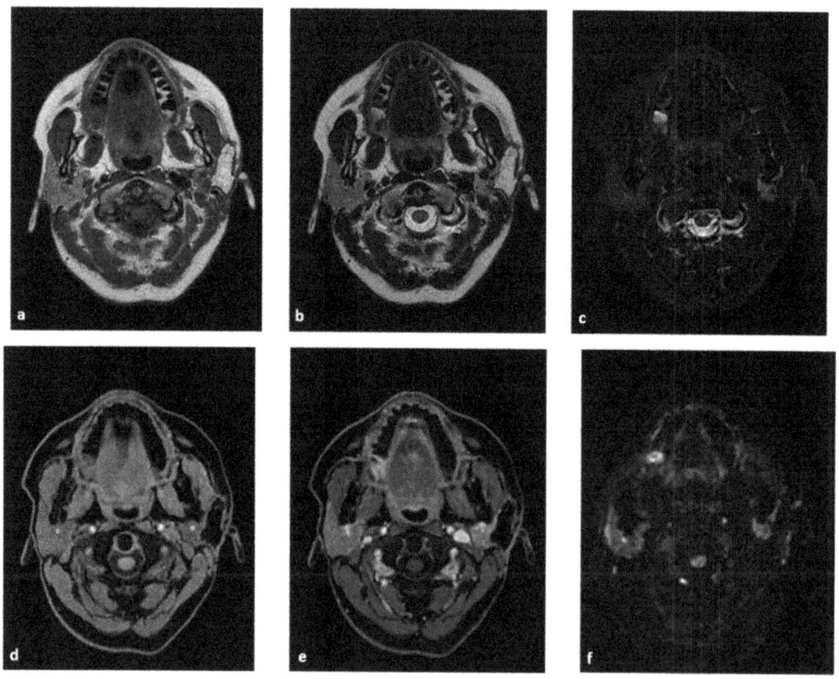

Figure 4. Female, 53 years old. First postoperative MR examination after partial parotidectomy with dermal fat graft. Fat appears hyperintense on both FSE T1-weighted (**a**) and T2-weighted (**b**) axial images and homogenously hypointense on STIR images (**c**). The fat graft shows no significant enhancement between pre- (**d**) and postcontrast (**e**) acquisitions and appears hypointense on DWI at b-1000 (**f**).

Differential diagnosis with tumour recurrence was also feasible, as the latter shows an intermediate T1-weighted signal and, most importantly, a variable degree of contrast enhancement and restricted diffusion.

The volumetric comparison conducted in postoperative studies showed no significant difference in volume between the two parotid glands (Figure 5).

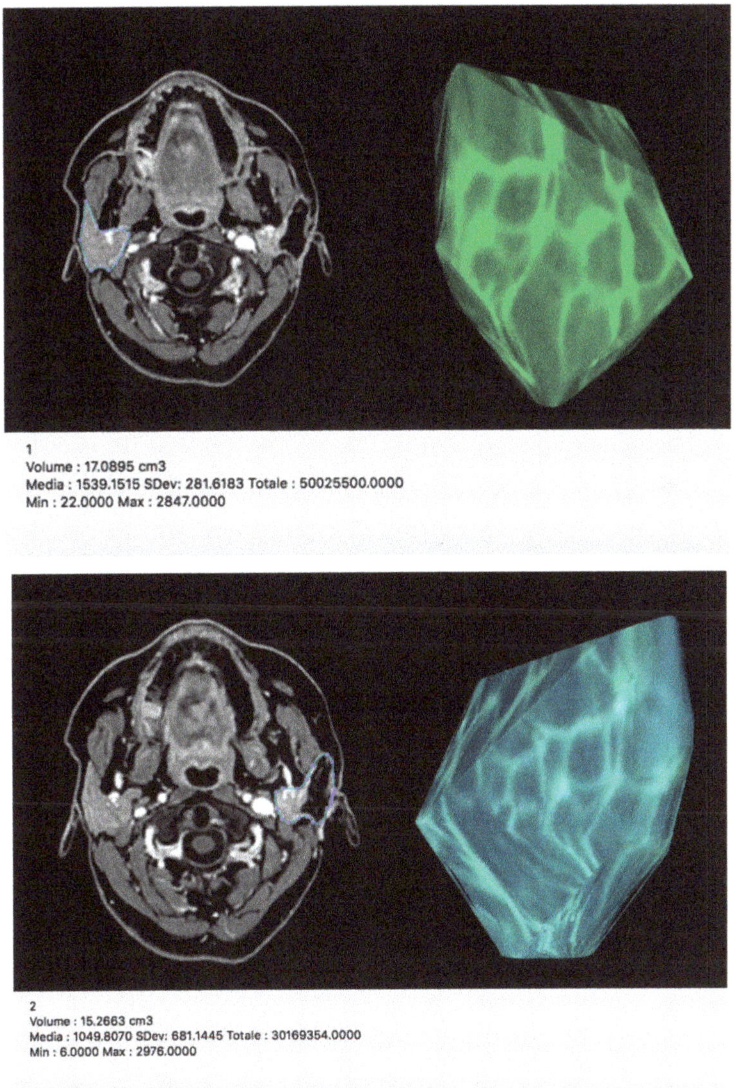

Figure 5. Postoperative volumetric comparison with 3D reconstruction between the contralateral (**1**) and the reconstructed parotid gland (**2**) shows minimal difference in volume (17.1 cm^3 vs. 15.2 cm^3).

5. Conclusions

Based on our satisfactory feedback received from patients about the overall postoperative cosmetic result, and with validation from our radiology team regarding the safety of this surgical procedure even in patients with malignant lesions, we can define fat grafting as a surgical procedure with high rates of success in terms of aesthetic results, the duration of the entire procedure, and its safety profile during the oncological follow up; with our experience, we confirm the already well-known fame of the autologous dermis-fat graft as a milestone in craniofacial reconstructive surgery.

Author Contributions: Conceptualization, C.E.B. and G.C.; methodology, G.T., M.S. and S.C.; software, M.P.B.; validation N.C.; formal analysis, G.C. and M.S.; investigation, R.V.; resources R.V.; data curation, S.C. and V.C.; writing—original draft preparation, R.V. and N.C.; writing—review and editing, G.T.; visualization, M.P.B.; supervision, G.C.; project administration, C.E.B. and R.V. All authors have read and agreed to the published version of the manuscript.

Funding: This research received no external funding.

Institutional Review Board Statement: This research received no external funding. The study was conducted in accordance with the Declaration of Helsinki. Our work was a retrospective study approved by the ethics committee of the University of Campania "Luigi Vanvitelli" (prot. 0013333, 29 April 2021).Institutional Review Board StatementThe study was conducted as a retrospective study; the study was approved by the ethics committee of the University of Campania "Luigi Vanvitelli" (prot. 0013333, 29 April 2021).

Informed Consent Statement: Patients' consent was obtained and can be produced on request. The study was conducted in accordance with the Declaration of Helsinki. Informed consent was obtained from all subjects involved in the study.

Data Availability Statement: Data are available upon reasonable request from the corresponding author (R.V.).

Conflicts of Interest: The authors declare no conflict of interest.

References

1. Wang, K.; Yang, Z.; Wang, W.; Xu, H.; Liu, F. Autologous Free Fat Graft for Repair of Concave Deformity after Total Parotidectomy. *J. Craniofac. Surg.* **2019**, *30*, 834–837. [CrossRef] [PubMed]
2. Kaufman, M.R.; Miller, T.A.; Huang, C.; Roostaien, J.; Wasson, K.L.; Ashley, R.K.; Bradley, J.P. Autologous fat transfer for facial recontouring: Is there science behind the art? *Plast. Reconstr. Surg.* **2007**, *119*, 2287–2296. [CrossRef] [PubMed]
3. Tunca, M.; Süslü, N.S.; Karaosmanoğlu, A.A. Fat Transfer after Parotidectomy: Fat Resorption Rates, Aesthetic and Functional Outcomes of En-Bloc Fat Graft Versus Lipofilling Technique. *Eur. Arch. Otorhinolaryngol.* **2021**, *278*, 3933–3940. [CrossRef] [PubMed]
4. Bryant, L.M.; Cognetti, D.; Baker, A.; Roy, S.; Johnston, D.R.; Curry, J.; Krein, H. Esthetic and functional reconstruction after parotidectomy in pediatric patients—A case series. *Int. J. Pediatr. Otorhinolaryngol.* **2015**, *79*, 2442–2445. [CrossRef]
5. Gir, P.; Brown, S.A.; Oni, G.; Kashefi, N.; Mojallal, A.; Rohrich, R.J. Fat Grafting. *Plast. Reconstr. Surg.* **2012**, *130*, 249–258. [CrossRef]
6. Brooker, J.E.; Rubin, J.P.; Marra, K.G. The Future of Facial Fat Grafting. *J. Craniofac. Surg.* **2019**, *30*, 644–651. [CrossRef]
7. Nofal, A.A.; Mohamed, M. Sternocleidomastoid Muscle Flap after Parotidectomy. *Int. Arch. Otorhinolaryngol.* **2015**, *19*, 319–324. [CrossRef]
8. Ambro, B.T.; Goodstein, L.A.; Morales, R.E.; Taylor, R.J. Evaluation of superficial musculoaponeurotic system flap and fat graft outcomes for benign and malignant parotid disease. *Otolaryngol. Head Neck Surg.* **2013**, *148*, 949–954. [CrossRef]
9. Irvine, L.E.; Larian, B.; Azizzadeh, B. Locoregional Parotid Reconstruction. *Otolaryngol. Clin. N. Am.* **2016**, *49*, 435–446. [CrossRef]
10. Keles, M.K.; Horoz, U.; Cepni, H. A simple method for breast de-epithelialization: The monobloc method. *Trichol. Cosmetol. Open J.* **2016**, *1*, 19–20. [CrossRef]
11. Boschetti, C.E.; Lo Giudice, G.; Spuntarelli, C.; Apice, C.; Rauso, R.; Santagata, M.; Tartaro, G.; Colella, G. Kabat Rehabilitation in Facial Nerve Palsy after Parotid Gland Tumor Surgery: A Case-Control Study. *Diagnostics* **2022**, *12*, 565. [CrossRef] [PubMed]
12. Garro, A.; Nigrovic, L.E. Managing Peripheral Facial Palsy. *Ann. Emerg. Med.* **2018**, *71*, 618–624. [CrossRef] [PubMed]
13. Conger, B.T.; Gourin, C.G. Free abdominal fat transfer for reconstruction of the total parotidectomy defect. *Laryngoscope* **2008**, *118*, 1186–1190. [CrossRef]
14. Guijarro-Martínez, R.; Alba, L.M.; Mateo, M.M.; Torres, M.P.; Gil, J.V.P. Autologous fat transfer to the cranio-maxillofacial region: Updates and controversies. *J. Craniomaxillofac. Surg.* **2011**, *39*, 359–363. [CrossRef]
15. Neuber, G. Fat transplantation. *Chir. Klongr. Verhandl. Dtsch. Gesellsch. Chir.* **1893**, *22*, 66.
16. De Cicco, D.; Tartaro, G.; Colella, G.; Dell'Aversana Orabona, G.; Santagata, M.; Ferrieri, I.; Troiano, A.; Staglianò, S.; Volgare, A.S.; D'Amato, S. Fat Graft in Surgical Treatment of Medication-Related Osteonecrosis of the Jaws (MRONJ). *Appl. Sci.* **2021**, *11*, 11195. [CrossRef]

17. Strong, A.L.; Cederna, P.S.; Rubin, J.P.; Coleman, S.R.; Levi, B. The Current State of Fat Grafting: A Review of Harvesting, Processing, and Injection Techniques. *Plast. Reconstr. Surg.* **2015**, *136*, 897–912. [CrossRef]
18. Colella, G.; Rauso, R.; De Cicco, D.; Boschetti, C.E.; Iorio, B.; Spuntarelli, C.; Franco, R.; Tartaro, G. Clinical management of squamous cell carcinoma of the tongue: Patients not eligible for free flaps, a systematic review of the literature. *Expert Rev. Anticancer. Ther.* **2021**, *21*, 9–22. [CrossRef]
19. Baum, S.; Prörtner, R.; Ladwein, F.; Schmeling, C.; Rieger, G.; Mohr, C. Use of dermis-fat grafts in the prevention of Frey's syndrome after parotidectomy. *J. Craniomaxillofac. Surg.* **2016**, *44*, 301–308. [CrossRef]
20. Chan, L.S.; Barakate, M.S.; Havas, T.E. Free fat grafting in superficial parotid surgery to prevent Frey-s syndrome and improve aesthetic outcome. *J. Laryngol. Otol.* **2014**, *128* (Suppl. S1), S44–S49. [CrossRef]
21. Boschetti, C.E.; Vitagliano, R.; Staglianò, S.; Pollice, A.; Giudice, G.L.; Apice, C.; Santagata, M.; Tartaro, G.; Colella, G. Development of an application for mobile phones (App) capable to predict the improvement of the degree House Brackmann scale in patients suffering from iatrogenic facial palsy. *Adv. Oral Maxillofac. Surg.* **2022**, *8*, 100356. [CrossRef]
22. Dehdashtian, A.; Bratley, J.V.; Svientek, S.R.; Kung, T.A.; Awan, T.M.; Cederna, P.S.; Kemp, S.W. Autologous fat grafting for nerve regeneration and neuropathic pain: Current state from bench-to-bedside. *Regen. Med.* **2020**, *15*, 2209–2228. [CrossRef] [PubMed]

Journal of
Personalized Medicine

MDPI

Article

Total Joint Replacement for Immediate Reconstruction following Ablative Surgery for Primary Tumors of the Temporo-Mandibular Joint

Luis-Miguel Gonzalez-Perez [1,2,*], Jose-Francisco Montes-Carmona [1], Eusebio Torres-Carranza [1] and Pedro Infante-Cossio [1,2]

1 Department of Oral and Maxillofacial Surgery, Virgen del Rocio University Hospital, 41013 Seville, Spain; josmoncar@gmail.com (J.-F.M.-C.); drtorres@clinicatorrescarranza.es (E.T.-C.); pinfante@us.es (P.I.-C.)
2 Department of Surgery, School of Medicine, University of Seville, 41009 Seville, Spain
* Correspondence: lumigon@telefonica.net

Abstract: Temporomandibular joint (TMJ) tumors are rare and difficult to diagnose. The purpose of this retrospective study was to evaluate the clinicopathologic characteristics of twenty-one patients with primary TMJ tumors between 2010 and 2019 and to analyze the surgical outcome and morbidity after ablative surgery and TMJ replacement. This case series confirmed the difficulty of diagnosis and reaffirmed the need for early recognition and management of TMJ tumors. There were no pathognomonic findings associated with TMJ tumors, although single or multiple radiopaque or radiolucent areas were observed on plain or panoramic radiographs. Occasionally, bone resorption or mottled densities caused by pathologic calcification and ossification were seen. Computed tomography and magnetic resonance imaging played an important role in the diagnosis. In our study, the distribution of histologic types of TMJ tumors was quite different from that of other joint tumors. The recommended treatment was surgical intervention by ablation of the joint and TMJ replacement. The results of this retrospective study support the surgical exeresis and replacement with TMJ stock and custom-made prostheses and show that the approach is efficacious and safe, reduces pain and improves mandibular movements, with few complications.

Keywords: temporomandibular joint; primary tumors; diagnosis; surgical treatment; temporo-mandibular joint replacement; joint prosthesis

1. Introduction

Primary tumors of the temporomandibular joint (TMJ) are not very common and often mimic common conditions, such as masticatory myalgia or internal derangement, leading to a delay in diagnosis and, therefore, to a delayed therapeutic option [1–8]. Radiographically, no pathognomonic findings are associated with TMJ tumors, although single or multiple radiolucent or radiopaque areas can be seen on plain or panoramic studies. Evidence of bone destruction is often present, and mottled densities caused by pathological calcification and ossification can occasionally be seen. Computed tomography (CT) and magnetic resonance imaging (MRI) play an important role in the diagnosis of these entities. The distribution of histological types of primary TMJ tumors is quite different from other articular tumors, with a predominance of benign histological forms. Their clinical presentation in the mandibular condyle usually consists of a combination of preauricular pain and impaired temporo-mandibular function with mandibular movement limitation, dentofacial deformity and occlusal asymmetry [9–15]. Resection and replacement of the TMJ is usually reserved for patients with irreversible damage, as in tumoral pathology [16–20].

The objective of this retrospective study was to investigate the clinical, radiological and histopathological characteristics of patients with primary TMJ tumors who were managed with ablative surgery and immediate reconstruction with total joint replacement and to evaluate their surgical outcome and morbidity.

2. Materials and Methods

Twenty-three patients with TMJ tumoral pathology were referred to the Department of Oral and Maxillofacial Surgery of the Virgen del Rocio University Hospital of Seville, Spain, between January 2010 and January 2019. The cases studied were adult male and female patients referred to the outpatient clinic with a primary TMJ tumor who were treated with ablative surgery and immediate reconstruction with total joint replacement. The following inclusion diagnostic criteria were assessed: (1) a history of persistent and significant pain and functional impairment; (2) a clinically and radiographically documented tumoral history. The exclusion criteria were: (1) patients without 5 years of follow-up, (2) infective disease at the implantation site, (3) insufficient quantity of bone support; (4) documented allergy of any of the prosthetic materials. Two patients, one with metastatic carcinoma and one with extraarticular location, were excluded from the study.

Twenty-one patients who met the inclusion criteria, nine males (43%) and twelve females (57%), were included in the study. All patients were initially investigated with plain radiographs. CT and/or MRI scans were performed in all the cases included in this study. Bone scintigraphy was performed in 4 cases. The mean preoperative period from initial TMJ symptoms to surgical treatment was 1 year (range: 6 months to 4 years).

The recommended treatment was surgical intervention by ablation of the joint and TMJ replacement. In all cases, surgical procedure was performed under general anesthesia with nasotracheal intubation. After the preauricular approach and the Al-Kayat–Bramley incision, a condylectomy was performed for the removal of the tumor. The glenoid fossa was then flattened, and the fossa was adapted and inserted. All surgeries were performed using the Zimmer Biomet Microfixation TMJ Replacement System®, Jacksonville, FL, USA (stock and custom-made prosthetic systems), and all procedures replaced the glenoid fossa component and the mandibular condyle. The fossa and mandibular components were available in three different sizes in the stock prosthetic system. The mandibular component of the prosthesis was manufactured from a cobalt–chromium–molybdenum (Co-Cr-Mb) alloy with a roughened titanium plasma coating on the host bone side of the ramal plate for increased bony integration. The Co-Cr-Mb alloy was type 99 of the American Society for Testing and Materials (ASTM). The fossa prosthesis was made of ultra-high-molecular-weight polyethylene (UHMWPE). In the stock TMJ replacement, templates were used intraoperatively to determine the fit, and then, the final TMJ prosthesis was inserted. The precision of a custom-made prosthesis makes the use of TMJ templates unnecessary. The screws used in the procedure were made of 6Al/4V titanium alloy. Intermaxillary fixation was temporary performed to restore the vertical dimension and dental occlusion. When the desired position was reached, the templates were replaced for the final prosthetic components.

The change in pain intensity (preoperative vs. current) was evaluated using a visual analog scale (VAS, 1 to 10), with higher scores indicating more severe pain. Jaw opening was measured in centimeters with a Therabite rule between incisal edges of maxillary central incisors. The signs assessed as indicators of the efficacy of surgical treatment were a significant reduction in pain at rest of 4 points or more, an improvement in temporomandibular function, and recovery of normal ranges of mandibular opening.

Active opening jaw motion initiated by patient's masticatory musculature was started immediately postoperatively. A soft food diet was recommended for the first month and normal sustenance thereafter. At follow-up, all patients were asked about any limitation in the activities of daily living and were examined for range of motion of TMJ or any neurovascular deficit. Imaging studies were carried out immediately after the operation and at 5-year follow-up for evaluation. All patients with TMJ tumors underwent radiological studies every 3 months during the first 2 years and every 6 months beginning the third postoperative year, and a CT scan was obtained in those with persistent symptoms or suspected recurrent TMJ lesions. Surgical morbidity and prosthetic implant survival were documented.

3. Results

The clinical, radiological and histopathological characteristics of the 21 patients are summarized in Table 1. The mean age was 54 years (range: 29–72 years). The main reasons for the consultation were mandibular deviation in 8 cases and posterior open bite in 7 cases (Figures 1–4). Less frequent were asymmetric prognathism (2 cases), preauricular swelling (2 cases) and TMJ dysfunction (2 cases). Radiologically, 13 cases presented as radiopaque lesions, 3 cases showed radiopaque areas, 2 cases radiolucent areas and 2 cases mottled densities. One case of bone destruction due to a malignant lesion (chondrosarcoma) was found.

Table 1. Clinical, radiological and histopathological characteristics of patients.

N°	Age/ Sex	Clinical Signs	Imaging Characteristics	Preop Pain *	5 yr Postop Pain *	Preop Opening **	5 yr Postop Opening **	Histological Diagnosis	Prosthesis Side
1	62/F	Mandibular deviation	Radiopaque lesion	4	0	2.5	3.5	Osteochondroma	Right
2	57//F	Posterior open bite	Radiopaque lesion	5	0	3	3	Osteochondroma	Left
3	57/M	Posterior open bite	Bone destruction	8	0	4.2	4.8	Chondrosarcoma	Right
4	60/F	Mandibular deviation	Radiopaque lesion	5	0	3.2	3.8	Osteochondroma	Left
5	49/M	Preauricular swelling	Radiopaque area	6	0	3.8	4.1	Osteochondroma	Right
6	67/F	Mandibular deviation	Radiopaque area	5	4	4	4	Osteoma	Right
7	65/F	Posterior open bite	Radiopaque area	7	2	3.5	3.7	Osteochondroma	Left
8	59/F	Asymmetric prognathism	Radiopaque lesion	4	0	4.2	4.5	Osteoma	Left
9	51/F	Posterior open bite	Radiopaque lesion	4.5	0	2.4	3.6	Osteochondroma	Right
10	59/F	Mandibular deviation	Radiopaque lesion	5	2	3.4	4.5	Osteoma	Left
11	52/M	TMJ dysfunction	Radiolucent areas	6	1	3.7	4.8	Osteochondroma	Bilateral
12	53/F	Preauricular swelling	Radiopaque lesion	6	2	3.1	3.6	Chondroblastoma	Left
13	68/M	Mandibular deviation	Radiolucent area	8	2	3.7	4.4	Osteochondroma	Left
14	30/F	TMJ dysfunction	Mottled densities	6	2	4.3	5	Osteochondroma	Right
15	48/M	Mandibular deviation	Mottled densities	5	0	4.8	5	Chondromyxoid fibroma	Right
16	55/F	Asymmetric prognathism	Radiopaque lesion	5	0	2.9	3.6	Osteochondroma	Left
17	38/M	Mandibular deviation	Radiopaque lesion	6	0	4.6	5.3	Osteochondroma	Left
18	56/M	Posterior cross-bite	Radiopaque lesion	6	1	4.1	4.1	Osteochondroma	Right
19	43/M	Posterior cross-bite	Radiopaque lesion	6	0	4	4.5	Osteochondroma	Bilateral
20	29/F	Posterior cross-bite	Radiopaque lesion	7	1	3.1	4.4	Osteochondroma	Bilateral
21	72/M	Mandibular deviation	Radiopaque lesion	7	3	2.7	3.5	Osteochondroma	Left

Abbreviations: M, male; F, female; Yr, years. * Pain intensity measured by VAS, Visual Analogue Scale. ** Mandibular opening measured in centimeters (cm). Preop, preoperative; Postop, postoperative.

After TMJ replacement, all the patients were followed up for at least 5 years (range: 5–10 years). Mean pain (VAS) and preoperative opening (cm) were 5.9 (range: 4–8) and 3.5 (range: 2.4–4.8), respectively. Mean pain (VAS) and postoperative opening (cm) measured at 5 years were 1 (range: 0–4) and 4.2 (range: 3–5.3), respectively. Therefore, a pain reduction of 4.9 points on the VAS scale and a postoperatively increased mouth opening of 0.7 cm were observed. Pain intensity was reduced by 83%. Jaw opening was improved by 20%.

Resection margins were wide in all cases (Figures 2 and 4). All diagnoses were confirmed by anatomopathological study. Most of the histopathological diagnoses were osteochondromas in 15 cases (71% of our studied population). Three cases were osteomas and one each of chondroblastoma, chondromyxoid fibroma and chondrosarcoma. A total of 24 joints (18 unilateral and 3 bilateral) were operated on, and consequently, 24 TMJ prostheses were fitted. All surgeries were performed with the Zimmer Biomet Microfixation

TMJ Replacement System®, Jacksonville, FL, USA, replacing both the skull base component (glenoid fossa) and the mandibular condyle. Twenty-two stock prostheses and two custom-made prostheses were implanted (Figures 5 and 6). Occlusal equilibration was required in one patient with persistent premature occlusal contacts. No particular predilection for tumor location within the TMJ was observed (left TMJ: 13 cases, right TMJ: 11 cases).

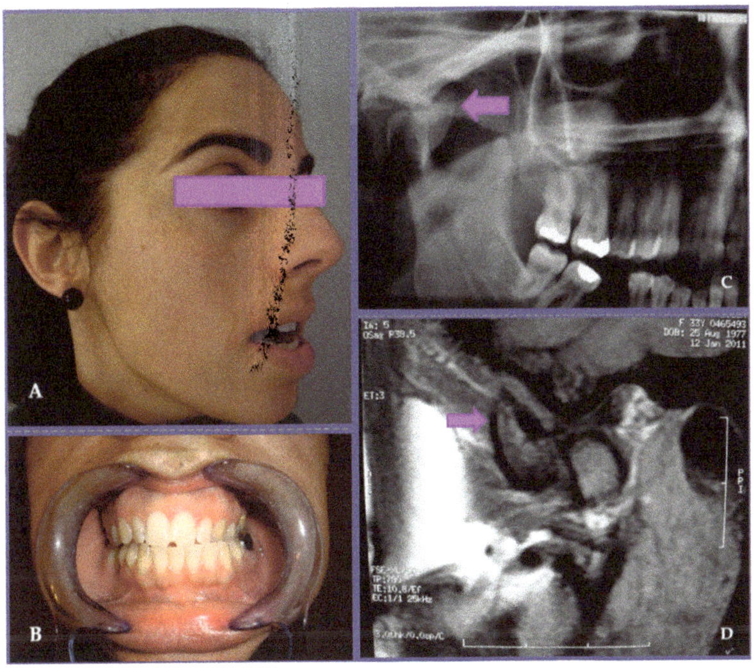

Figure 1. Osteochondroma is one of the most common benign tumors of the axial skeleton but is rarely found in the TMJ. (**A**) Its clinical presentation in the mandibular condyle, as in our 5th case, usually occurs with a combination of preauricular pain, mandibular dysfunction and facial asymmetry. When considering surgical risks involved in tumoral exeresis and temporomandibular reconstruction, the differential diagnosis is of great importance. (**B**) In this patient, an osteochondroma was suspected given the clinical characteristics of the lesion; restricted mouth opening and changes in occlusion with unilateral posterior open bite and contralateral crossbite were related to the anatomical location of the tumor and were due to alterations in the vertical dimension. Orthopantomography (**C**) and magnetic resonance imaging (**D**) showed an osteochondroma with growth arising from the anterolateral aspect of the right mandibular condyle (see arrows), distinguishing it from condylar hyperplasia, seen as an enlargement of the condylar process.

Comparing stock and customized groups, no statistically significant differences were detected with respect to reduction in pain intensity and improvement in maximum mouth opening compared, although these data should be considered carefully given the small number of cases in the customized prostheses group.

Functional and oncological results of the surgery were good. No patient reported 7th nerve dysfunction after 3 months. Two of twenty-four implants (TMJ prostheses) were explanted during the study period of 10 years, as a result of instability of the implant for screw loosening and metal hypersensitivity. The patient's satisfaction with the clinical outcome was 9 on a scale of 1 to 10. Recurrence has not been reported in our patients.

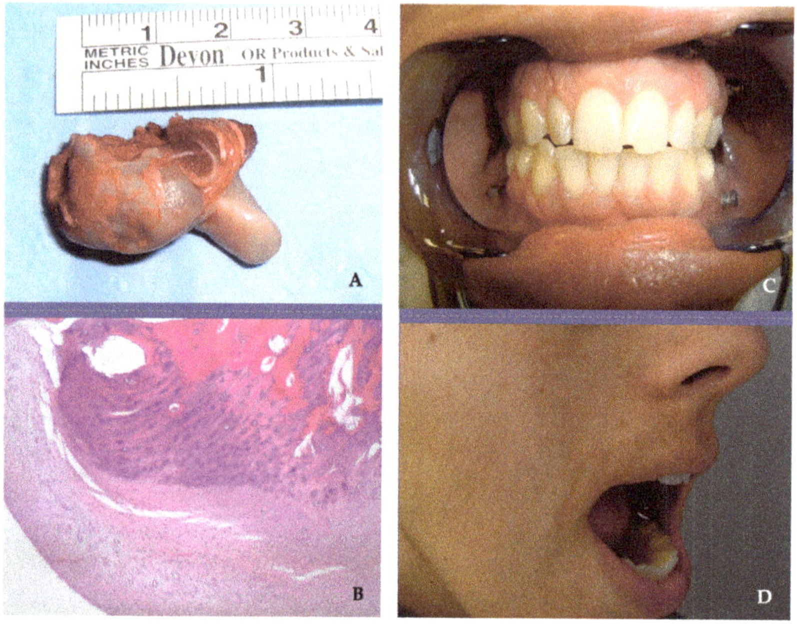

Figure 2. (**A**) Surgical resection of clinical case shown in Figure 1. The tumor showed no infiltration of the surrounding tissues. (**B**) Histopathological diagnosis was osteochondroma. (**C**,**D**) Postoperative view of the patient shows correction of the occlusal alterations and increased mouth opening after surgery.

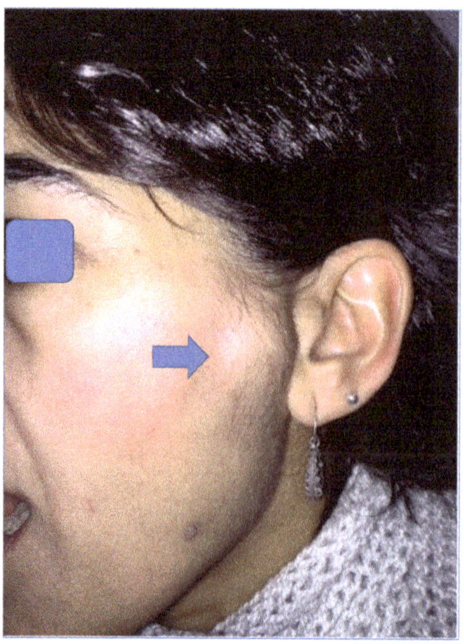

Figure 3. Painful and slow-growing TMJ osteochondroma in the left preauricular area (see arrow), with facial asymmetry, accompanied by ipsilateral open bite and right mandibular lateral deviation in our patient (case number 17).

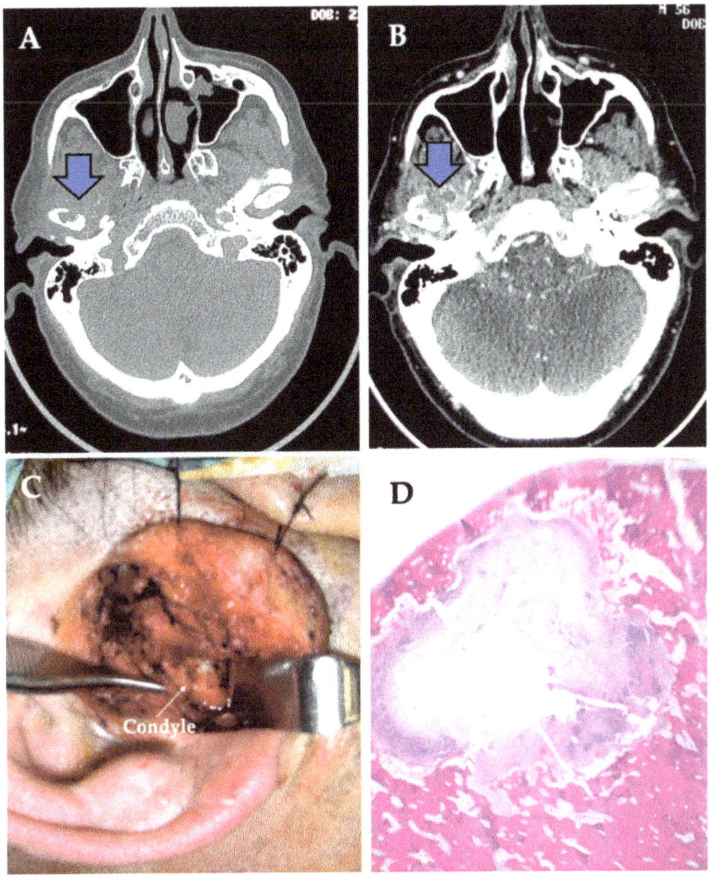

Figure 4. (**A**,**B**) Computed tomography, without and with contrast, shows well-delimited lytic lesion involving right mandibular condyle (see arrows), and is recommended as the imaging study of choice when planning a surgical treatment. (**C**) The TMJ tumor appeared well encapsulated with an expansile intramedullary lesion (see arrow). The surgical TMJ defect was replaced with a total prosthesis. (**D**) The tumor in the condylar specimen was whitish and hard elastic with a central cavitation. The margins of surgical resection appeared without tumor. There was no extraosseous infiltration. The histopathological diagnosis was of primary intramedullary chondrosarcoma (case number 3).

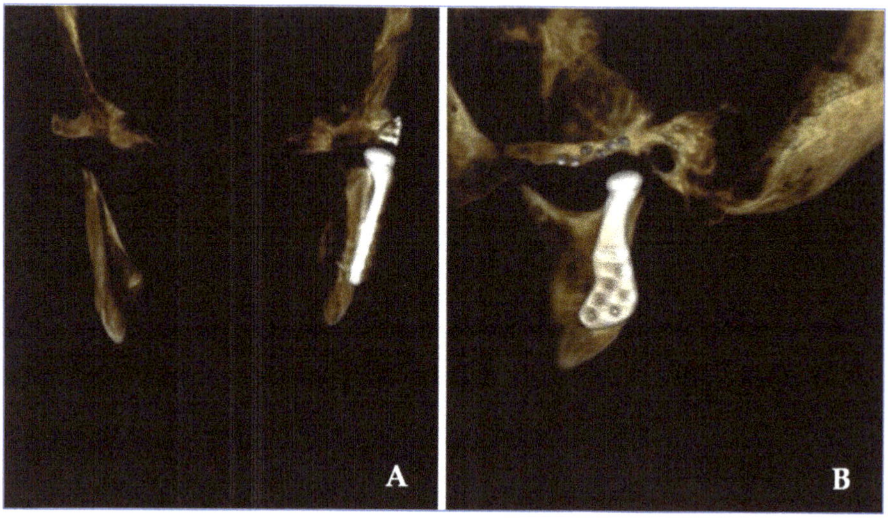

Figure 5. Postoperative tridimensional computed tomography reconstruction of clinical case shown in Figure 3. (**A**) Coronal view. (**B**) Sagittal view.

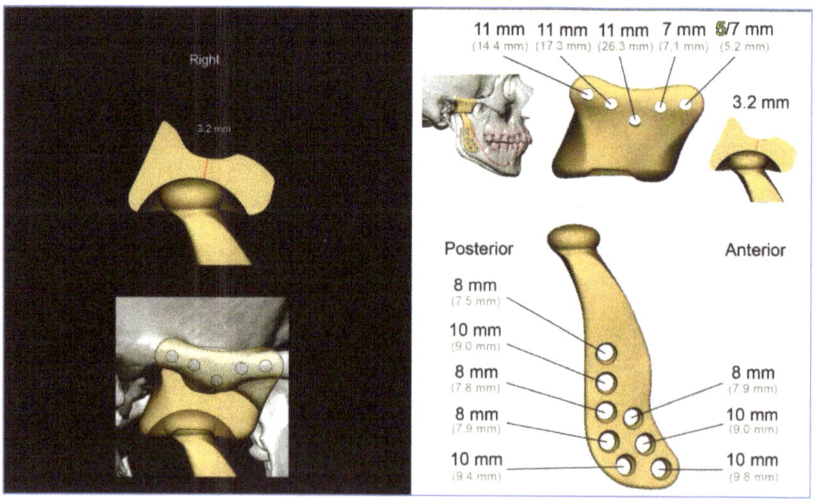

Figure 6. Custom-made prosthesis, designed for one of our cases, using the patient's DICOM data.

4. Discussion

The temporomandibular joint (TMJ) is one of the most complex and widely used joints and is the only paired joint of the skeletal system. The most frequent pathologies of the TMJ are dysfunctional disorders, internal derangement, masticatory myalgias and degenerative arthropathies, which cause considerable structural and functional abnormalities leading to early diagnosis. Primary tumors of the TMJ are rare and represent a diagnostic enigma due to their non-specific clinical course and radiographic presentation. There is little literature available on their characteristics and outcomes; thus, experience in the treatment of tumors and tumoral lesions in this anatomical area is limited. There are several types of tumors that can affect the TMJ, as any other joint, including benign tumors, such as osteochondroma (Figures 1–3), osteoma, osteoblastoma, chondroma, chondroblastoma, non-ossifying fibroma, hemangioma or lipoma, as well as malignant tumors such as synovial sarcoma, osteosarcoma, Ewing sarcoma or chondrosarcoma (Figure 4) [1,2,5,9,11, 21–31]. The wide variety of primary tumors of the TMJ indicates the great range of possible treatments, with most of them based on surgical intervention (Table 2).

Table 2. Primary tumors of the temporo-mandibular joint classification.

	Benign	Aggressive	Malignant
Bone formers	Osteoid osteoma Osteoma	Osteoblastoma	Osteosarcoma
Cartilage formers	Osteochondroma Chondroma (enchondroma and periosteal chondroma)	Chondroblastoma	Chondrosarcoma Osteochondrosarcoma Synovial sarcoma
Fibrous tissue formers	Chondromyxoid fibroma	Desmoid (aggressive fibromatosis)	Malignant fibrous histiocytoma Fibrosarcoma
Round cell			Ewing's sarcoma Primitive neuroectodermal tumor
Myelogenous		Eosinophilic granuloma (histiocytosis X, Langerhans cells)	Myeloma Solitary plasmacytoma Reticulosarcoma (bone malignant lymphoma)
Lipogenic	Lipoma		Liposarcoma
Myogenic			Leiomyosarcoma Rhabdomyosarcoma
Vascular	Hemangioma		Angiosarcoma
Neurogenic	Neurilemmoma		
Unfilial lineage		Giant cell tumor	Chordoma Adamantinoma
Pseudotumoral lesions	Non-ossifying fibroma Cortical fibrous defect Essential bone cyst Aneurysmal bone cyst Fibrous dysplasia Bone infarction Myositis ossificans Brown tumor of hyperparathyroidism	Osteomyelitis Paget's disease Pigmented villonodular synovitis Synovial chondromatosis	

The classification of TMJ tumors plays a key role in the understanding, diagnosis, and treatment of these rare clinical conditions. Since these tumors can present with a wide variety of histological and clinical characteristics, their classification is essential to establish a multidisciplinary and collaborative approach in clinical practice between maxillofacial surgeons, pathologists, radiologists, and oncologists, and it is essential to ensure optimal management of these complex cases (Table 2).

In our study, osteochondroma was the most common neoplasm affecting the TMJ [3,4,7,11–15]. Osteochondroma is one of the most common benign tumors of the axial skeleton but is rarely found in the TMJ. Its clinical presentation is in the mandibular condyle, as observed in our case series. Primary TMJ tumors are rare lesions with a histopathological profile quite different from that seen in other articular areas, and they often mimic common conditions of the TMJ, such as TMJ dysfunctional syndrome and neurologic or otologic pathologies, leading to a delay in diagnosis and surgical treatment. For this reason, a high index of suspicion is needed for the timely diagnosis and management of tumors at this rare site. This may lead to earlier intervention and may improve outcome [3–5,7–10,12–15,21,23,27]. In some patients, benign tumors of the TMJ remain as totally asymptomatic lesions. In patients who have intense pain that does not respond to conservative treatment for more than one year, radiographic imaging may be considered to rule out these tumors. Changes in occlusion with ipsilateral posterior open bite and contralateral posterior crossbite are related to the anatomical location of the tumors and are due to alterations in the vertical dimension (Figures 1 and 3). These occlusal disorders disappeared after surgical treatment (Figure 2). Considering the surgical risks involved in tumor removal and temporomandibular reconstruction, prior differential diagnosis was of great importance. In our cases, osteochondroma was suspected given the clinical characteristics of the lesion. The changes in occlusion with unilateral posterior open bite and contralateral crossbite were related to the anatomical location of the tumor and were due to the alteration of the vertical dimension [4–6,10–27].

Surgical treatment of TMJ tumors depends on several factors such as the type, size, location, and extent of the tumor, as well as the patient's overall health and individual circumstances. In general, surgical treatment involves the removal of the tumor as well as any affected surrounding tissue. The goal of surgery is to completely remove the tumoral lesion while minimizing damage to the surrounding structures of the mandible and other facial structures. Treatment of TMJ tumors should mostly include partial or complete resection, the oncological and functional results of which are good [2–7,10,11,14,15,31]. In our series, which had a relatively large number of cases and a minimum follow-up of 5 years, there were no recurrences. Immediate reconstruction after resection of a primary TMJ tumor is a good strategy to avoid a second operation.

The visual analogue scale (VAS) on pain was measured at rest in our analysis. TMJ pain in end-stage TMJ disease is often a dull, constant and severe long-standing ache that is aggravated, in a very variable way according to the patients, by mandibular opening or mastication. There is usually a complaint of reduced jaw mobility preoperatively and frequent grinding noise within the TMJ associated with mandibular movement or chewing. The reason for our results in jaw opening is that although none of the surgical procedures were carried out in patients who had good mandibular motion, six patients included in the tumoral group (28% of 21 patients) had a preoperative normal mouth opening $\geq$4 cm, and although strictly speaking, there was no limited mouth opening, all of them were cases with a history of progressive mandibular deviation, open bite on the ipsilateral side and posterior crossbite on the contralateral side.

In our study, primary malignant tumors of the TMJ were unusual. They can invade sensory and motor nerves, causing paresthesia and paralysis in the TMJ area, mandible and lower lip. The eighth cranial nerve may be involved; thus, changes in hearing, tinnitus, or dizziness should be monitored. Changes in mandibular function are common, as in case number 3 in our study (Figure 4); thus, any abrupt change in occlusion, trismus, and pathologic fractures should be considered as a sign of malignancy. Pain is not a symptom indicative of malignant neoplasm, but it may occur in this TMJ area as an extension of other tumors, easily confused with myofascial pain syndrome and TMJ internal disorders, which in many cases have hindered early diagnosis of malignant disease. The most common, but outside the scope of our study, are metastatic tumors of the breast, lung, thyroid, prostate, stomach, skin, ovaries, colon and kidney, although maxillofacial, nasopharyngeal, and intracranial tumors that may metastasize to the TMJ should also be considered [5,9].

Primary intrinsic malignancies of the TMJ include chondrosarcoma (only one out of all our cases), osteosarcoma, osteochondrosarcoma, synovial sarcoma, fibrosarcoma and epidermoid carcinoma. Other tumors described with condylar involvement include multiple myeloma, solitary plasmacytoma or reticulosarcoma (bone malignant lymphoma). Chondrosarcoma, which usually occurs primarily in the long bones, presents as a rapidly growing asymptomatic form in the preauricular area. Pain, when it occurs, is caused by compression of the adjacent anatomical structures [5,9].

The management of TMJ reconstruction after ablative tumor surgery remains a challenge. In some cases, reconstructive surgery may be necessary to repair any damage to the mandible or craniofacial structures caused by the tumor or by surgery. This may involve the use of bone grafts or other materials to restore the temporo-mandibular structure and function. Surgery is often considered as an option of last resort. However, there are instances where surgery is the definitive and sometimes only treatment option. TMJ specialists must be prepared to recognize and manage disorders that present with more complex cases where TMJ surgery is less clear. While the diagnosis and surgical aims of severe tumoral cases are straight forward, when it comes to initial cases, the diagnosis is often complicated, and the surgical perspective is less clearly defined, especially when TMJ disease progression is slow. However, it can ultimately lead to end-stage TMJ disease with, as a consequence, significant disability requiring surgical intervention, as occurs in patients of this study [3,7,8,10,12,13,15–17,19–23,28–30].

To the best of our knowledge, the main surgical indication for a total TMJ prosthesis is the presence of a symptomatic severely damaged TMJ with extensive joint destruction (when nothing is salvageable), which can result from either different types of severe TMJ tumor disease or failed previous surgeries, and therefore, it is wrong not to consider surgical definitive treatment modality of collapsed articular cartilage and degenerative changes that severely interfere with the smooth, painless movement of the TMJ. When compared to other surgical reconstructive procedures, such as costochondral or sternoclavicular grafts, the use of TMJ prosthesis can reduce the duration of surgery and hospitalization time, which provides immediate function without intermaxillary fixation postoperatively and no morbidity from a donor site. The prosthetic replacement may also present some disadvantages such as loss of protrusion and laterality movements due to the detachment of the lateral pterygoid muscle during surgery, fracture of the TMJ prosthesis from metal fatigue, loosening of screws, etc. [12,15,20].

The surgical placement of TMJ prostheses, as it happened in our cases, provides significant reduction in pain intensity and secondary TMJ dysfunction to tumoral pathology of the TMJ (Figures 5 and 6). The appropriate selection of the case is the most important requirement for a successful surgical intervention to achieve the desired outcomes of relief of symptoms and improved function [3,4,7,10–15,17,19]. In our case series, the functional and oncological results of surgery were good.

The quantification of implant failures is a determining factor with prognostic value, enabling the clinician to objectively quantify the success of the surgical treatment [3,7,8,10,12,13,15–17,19–23]. Although there were complications necessitating the removal of the prosthesis (2 out of 24 prostheses: 8% of our studied population), there were no device-related mechanical failures; and one case of TMJ prosthesis was explanted due to malocclusion, which was a result of loosening of the implant screws. Another case was explanted due to severe hypersensitivity to the metal alloy not detected before surgical replacement, with only the mandibular prosthetic component replaced. Many factors contribute to the success or failure of a total TMJ replacement. These factors include prosthesis micromovements, loosening of prosthetic components, allergic reaction and metal hypersensitivity, material wear breakdown and corrosion, bacterial contamination, and the development of heterotopic bone apposition around the prosthesis [3,5,8,10,12,22,28]. In our series, only two prostheses had to be removed, even though the result was satisfactory for patients.

Two types of prosthetic implants were used in our study: stock TMJ replacement in which the surgeon must fit it to the implantation area, as occurred in 19 of our patients, and custom-made prostheses, which are made specifically for each clinical case, as had occurred in two of our patients.

The stock TMJ replacement must be compatible with a range of different patient geometries and anatomies, and typically a range of different sizes is necessary, such as large (55 mm), medium (50 mm) and small (45 mm) condyle–ramus components. Mainly, implant failure was a consequence of wear. The biomaterials from which prosthetic implants are made must be biocompatible, and any wear particles produced must be compatible with the body and must not cause adverse biological reactions, but the wear of materials is unpredictable. Similarly, the bone quality of patients varies considerably, and the methods of fixation must be able to accommodate different bone interface conditions [10,14,15,17,19,20,22].

One problem in planning surgery is the inability to predictably create complex prosthetic contours using commercially available stock prostheses. These devices are supplied as generic sizes and shapes designed on the basis of the average patient. In more complex and severe clinical cases, the surgeon may need prolonged operative time shaping the prosthesis to customize the stock prosthesis to fit the patient's bone contours, and these repeated manipulations to adapt the prosthesis to difficult anatomical conditions may cause prosthetic fracture due to material fatigue. One solution to this deficiency is to use computer-guided surgical planning technologies to create a passive fitting replacement designed for specific anatomical requirements. To date, the most common application of additive manufacturing has been the fabrication of patient-specific models (Figure 6), which are created for pre-operative planning using patient-specific imaging data in DICOM files (Digital Imaging/Communications in Medicine), which are then converted into stereolithography files, the standard manufacturing format used to print patient-specific cranio-facial models. The use of these medical models enables planning and simulation of surgery and manually pre-shapes commercially available prostheses. Recent advances in additive manufacturing allow for the prefabrication of patient-specific customized prostheses using the patient's DICOM data. The advantages of rapid prototyping in designing and manufacturing customized prostheses are that they do not require intraoperative modifications, and they provide a better passive fitting.

Considering the implanted material, which may invoke a tissue response, the materials used remain basically the same as before, namely, metal alloys and polymers (mostly polyethylene). Bioactive coatings and particulate materials constitute the last broad category to which the body reacts in joint replacement. Employing the most advantageous characteristics of biocompatible materials is an essential consideration in the design and manufacturing of any replacement device. In our cases, cobalt chromium alloy, with its undersurface coated with a roughened titanium plasma spray for increased osteointegration, contributes to its strength and biocompatibility. Its excellent wear characteristics when articulated against a UHMWPE material presently make it the standard for the non-moveable articulating surface of most orthopedic total joint replacement devices [12,15,17,19,20] (Figures 5 and 6).

The results of this case series support the need for further research breakdown of this form of surgical treatment in a rigorously controlled prospective analysis. Despite the fact that this case series includes a relatively high number of cases, the results should be taken with caution, and further long-term follow-up studies with clear results are still needed.

5. Conclusions

This was a retrospective study in a single center. The relatively large number of patients operated on and the standard operative and perioperative management made our study consistent and facilitated comparison with other studies. Temporomandibular joint (TMJ) tumors are rare lesions, with a histopathological profile quite different from that seen in other maxillofacial areas, and they often mimic common TMJ conditions, resulting in delayed diagnosis. There is often a long delay between the onset of initial symptoms and definitive diagnosis. A high index of suspicion is needed for timely diagnosis and treatment of tumors in these rare areas by integrating the components of patient history, clinical presentation, and imaging findings. This may lead to earlier intervention and a better outcome. Osteochondroma is the most common tumor in the TMJ. Changes in occlusion with ipsilateral posterior open bite and contralateral posterior crossbite are related to the anatomic location of the tumors and are due to alterations in the vertical dimension. These occlusal disorders disappeared after surgical treatment. Treatment of TMJ tumors should mostly include partial or complete resection, the oncological and functional results of which are good. The surgical placement of TMJ prostheses provides a significant reduction in pain intensity and TMJ dysfunction secondary to tumoral pathology of the TMJ. In our study, the main indication was a damaged TMJ with extensive destruction, which was the consequence of different tumors. When compared to other surgical reconstructive procedures, such as costochondral or sternoclavicular grafts, the use of a TMJ prosthesis can reduce the duration of surgery and hospitalization time and provides immediate function and no morbidity from a donor site. TMJ replacement is often considered to be the last resort in the surgical treatment of TMJ disorders and can be recognized as the gold standard treatment in immediate reconstruction after ablative surgery for primary tumors of TMJ.

Author Contributions: Conceptualization, L.-M.G.-P., J.-F.M.-C., E.T.-C. and P.I.-C.; methodology, L.-M.G.-P.; software, J.-F.M.-C., E.T.-C. and P.I.-C.; validation, L.-M.G.-P., J.-F.M.-C., E.T.-C. and P.I.-C.; formal analysis, L.-M.G.-P., J.-F.M.-C., E.T.-C. and P.I.-C.; investigation, L.-M.G.-P.; resources, L.-M.G.-P., J.-F.M.-C., E.T.-C. and P.I.-C.; data curation, L.-M.G.-P.; writing—original draft preparation, L.-M.G.-P., J.-F.M.-C., E.T.-C. and P.I.-C.; writing—review and editing, L.-M.G.-P., J.-F.M.-C., E.T.-C. and P.I.-C.; visualization, L.-M.G.-P., J.-F.M.-C., E.T.-C. and P.I.-C.; supervision, L.-M.G.-P.; project administration, L.-M.G.-P.; funding acquisition, L.-M.G.-P. All authors have read and agreed to the published version of the manuscript.

Funding: This study received no external funding.

Institutional Review Board Statement: This study was approved by the Research and Clinical Ethics Committee of Virgen del Rocio University Hospital, Seville, Spain (IRB number 2014PI/083). The Declaration of Helsinki guidelines were followed.

Informed Consent Statement: Written informed consent was obtained from all subjects involved in the study.

Data Availability Statement: The data presented in this study are available by contacting the corresponding author upon reasonable request.

Conflicts of Interest: The authors declare no conflict of interest.

References

1. Choi, J.H.; Ro, J.Y. The 2020 WHO Classification of Tumors of Bone: An Updated Review. *Adv. Anat. Patol.* **2021**, *28*, 119–138. [CrossRef]
2. Al Hayek, M.; Yousfan, A. Monophasic synovial sarcoma in the temporomandibular joint region: A case report and review of the literature. *Int. J. Surg. Case Rep.* **2023**, *105*, 107998. [CrossRef]
3. Gerbino, G.; Segura-Palleres, I.; Ramieri, G. Osteochondroma of the mandibular condyle: Indications for different surgical methods: A case series of 7 patients. *J. Craniomaxillofac. Surg.* **2021**, *49*, 584–591. [CrossRef] [PubMed]
4. Holmlund, A.B.; Gynther, G.W.; Reinholt, F.P. Surgical treatment of osteochondroma of the mandibular condyle in the adult: A 5-year follow-up. *Int. J. Oral Maxillofac. Surg.* **2004**, *33*, 549–553. [CrossRef]
5. Gonzalez-Perez, L.M.; Sanchez-Gallego, F.; Perez-Ceballos, J.L.; Lopez-Vaquero, D. Temporomandibular joint chondrosarcoma: Case report. *J. Craniomaxillofac. Surg.* **2011**, *39*, 79–83. [CrossRef] [PubMed]
6. Yu, H.B.; Sun, H.; Li, B.; Zhao, Z.L.; Zhang, L.; Shen, S.G. Endoscope-assisted conservative condylectomy in the treatment of condilar osteochondroma through an intraoral approach. *Int. J. Oral Maxillofac. Surg.* **2013**, *42*, 1582–1586. [CrossRef] [PubMed]
7. Ord, R.A.; Warburton, G.; Caccamese, J.F. Osteochondroma of the condyle: Review of 8 cases. *Int. J. Oral Maxillofac. Surg.* **2010**, *39*, 523–528. [CrossRef] [PubMed]
8. Liu, X.; Wan, S.; Abdelherem, A.; Chen, M.; Yang, C. Benign temporomandibular joint tumours with extension tio infratemporal fossa and skull base: Condyle preserving approach. *Int. J. Oral Maxillofac. Surg.* **2020**, *49*, 867–873. [CrossRef] [PubMed]
9. Faro, T.F.; Martins-de-Barros, A.V.; Fernandes Lima, G.T.W.; Pereira Raposo, A.; de Alburquerque Borges, M.; da Costa Araujo, F.A. Chondrosarcoma of the Temporomandibular Joint: Systematic Review and Survival Analysis of Cases Reported to Date. *Head Neck Pathol.* **2021**, *15*, 923–934. [CrossRef]
10. Bredell, M.; Gratz, K.; Obwegeser, J.; Gujer, A.K. Management of the Temporomandibular Joint after Ablative Surgery. *Craniomaxillofac. Trauma Reconstr.* **2014**, *7*, 271–279. [CrossRef]
11. Poveda-Roda, R.; Bagan, J.V.; Sanchis, J.M.; Margaix, M. Pseudotumors and tumors of the temporomandibular joint. A review. *Med. Oral Patol. Oral Cir. Bucal* **2013**, *18*, 392–402. [CrossRef] [PubMed]
12. Gonzalez-Perez, L.M.; Gonzalez-Perez-Somarriba, B.; Centeno, G.; Vallellano, C.; Montes-Carmona, J.F.; Torres-Carranza, E.; Ambrosiani-Fernandez, J.; Infante-Cossio, P. Prospective study of five-year outcomes and postoperative complications after total temporomandibular joint replacement with two stock prosthetic systems. *Br. J. Oral Maxillofac. Surg.* **2020**, *58*, 69–74. [CrossRef]
13. Morey-Mas, M.A.; Caubet-Biayna, J.; Iriarte-Ortabe, J.I. Osteochondroma of the Temporomandibular Joint Treated by Means of Condylectomy and Immediate Reconstruction with a Total Stock Prosthesis. *J. Oral Maxillofac. Res.* **2010**, *1*, e4. [CrossRef] [PubMed]
14. Kumar, V.V. Large osteochondroma of the mandibular condyle treated by condylectomy using a transzygomatic approach. *Int. J. Oral Maxillofac. Surg.* **2010**, *39*, 188–191. [CrossRef] [PubMed]
15. Park, J.H.; Jo, E.; Cho, H.; Kim, H.J. Temporomandibular joint reconstruction with alloplastic prosthesis: The outcomes of four cases. *Maxillofac. Plastic Reconst. Surg.* **2017**, *39*, 6. [CrossRef]
16. Peroz, I. Osteochondroma of the condyle: Case report with 15 years of follow-up. *Int. J. Oral Maxillofac. Surg.* **2016**, *45*, 1120–1122. [CrossRef]
17. Pedersen, T.O.; Lybak, S.; Lund, B.; Loes, S. Temporomandibular joint prosthesis in cancer reconstruction preceding radiation therapy. *Clin. Case Rep.* **2021**, *9*, 1438–1441. [CrossRef]

18. Graziano, P.; Spinzia, A.; Abbate, A.; Romano, A. Intra-articular loose osteochondroma of the temporomandibular joint. *Int. J. Oral Maxillofac. Surg.* **2012**, *41*, 1505–1508. [CrossRef]
19. Yaseen, M.; Abdulqader, D.; Audi, K.; Ng, M.; Audi, S.; Vaderhobil, R.M. Temporomandibular Total Joint Replacement Implant Devices: A Systematic Review of Their Outcomes. *J. Long. Term. Eff. Med. Implant.* **2021**, *31*, 91–98. [CrossRef]
20. Peres-Lima, F.G.G.; Rios, L.G.C.; Bianchi, J.; Goncalvez, J.R.; Paranhos, L.R.; Vieira, W.A.; Zanetta-Barbosa, D. Complications of total temporomandibular joint replacement: A systematic review and meta-analysis. *Int. J. Oral Maxillofac. Surg.* **2023**, *52*, 584–594. [CrossRef]
21. Mohapatra, M.; Banushree, C.S. Osteochondroma condyle: A journey of 20 years in a 52-year-old male patient causing severe facial asymmetry and occlusal derangement. *J. Oral Maxillofac. Pathol.* **2019**, *23*, 162. [CrossRef]
22. Mehra, P.; Arya, V.; Henry, C. Temporomandibular Joint Condylar Osteochondroma: Complete Condylectomy and Joint Replacement versus Low Condylectomy and Joint Preservation. *J. Oral Maxillofac. Surg.* **2016**, *74*, 911–925. [CrossRef]
23. Martinovic Guzman, G.; Carmona Avendaño, A.P.; Rueda Lama, C.; Plaza Alvarez, C. Osteochondroma of Mandibular Ramus and Condylar Neck: Simultaneous Resection and Reconstruction with Personalized Alloplastic Joint Prosthesis. *Int. J. Odontostomatol.* **2020**, *14*, 363–366. [CrossRef]
24. Arora, P.; Deora, S.S.; Kiran, S.; Bargale, S.D. Osteochondroma of condyle: Case discussion and review of treatment modalities. *BMJ Case Rep.* **2014**, *2014*, bcr2013200759. [CrossRef]
25. Lund, B.; Kruger Weiner, C.; Benchimol, D.; Holmlund, A. Osteochondroma of the glenoid fossa- report of two cases with sudden onset of symptoms. *Int. J. Oral Maxillofac. Surg.* **2014**, *43*, 1473–1476. [CrossRef]
26. Zhu, Z.; He, Z.; Tai, Y.; Liu, Y.; Liu, H.; Luo, E. Surgical Guides and Prebent Titanium Improve the Planning for the Treatment of Dentofacial Deformities Secondary to Condylar Osteochondroma. *J. Craniofac. Surg.* **2022**, *33*, 1488–1492. [CrossRef]
27. Mahajan, A.; Patil, D.J.; Shah, V.; Mulay, M. Giant Osteochondroma of the mandibular condyle and temporomandibular joint—A case report. *J. Oral Maxillofac. Pathol.* **2022**, *26*, 290–293.
28. Renno, T.A.; Chung, A.C.; Gitt, H.A.; Correa, L.; Luz, J.G. Temporomandibular arthropathies: A retrospective study with histopathological characteristics. *Med. Oral Patol. Oral Cir. Bucal.* **2019**, *24*, 562–570. [CrossRef] [PubMed]
29. Mercuri, L.G.; Saltzman, B.M. Acquired heterotopic ossification of the temporomandibular joint. *Int. J. Oral Maxillofac. Surg.* **2017**, *46*, 1562–1568. [CrossRef] [PubMed]
30. Dimitroulis, G. Comparison of the outcomes of three surgical treatments for end-stage temporomandibular joint disease. *Int. J. Oral Maxillofac. Surg.* **2014**, *43*, 980–989. [CrossRef] [PubMed]
31. Yang, X.; Wang, M.; Gao, W.; Wan, D.; Zheng, J.; Zhang, Z. Chondroblastoma of mandibular condyle: Case report and literature review. *Open Med.* **2021**, *16*, 1372–1377. [CrossRef] [PubMed]

Journal of *Personalized Medicine*

MDPI

Article

Airway Management of Orofacial Infections Originating in the Mandible

Andreas Sakkas [1,2,*], Christel Weiß [3], Wolfgang Zink [4], Camila Alejandra Rodriguez [5], Mario Scheurer [2], Sebastian Pietzka [1,2], Frank Wilde [1,2], Oliver Christian Thiele [6], Robert Andreas Mischkowski [6] and Marcel Ebeling [2]

1 Department of Cranio-Maxillo-Facial-Surgery, University Hospital Ulm, 89081 Ulm, Germany
2 Department of Cranio-Maxillo-Facial-Surgery, German Armed Forces Hospital Ulm, 89081 Ulm, Germany
3 Medical Statistics and Biomathematics, Mannheim Medical Faculty of the Heidelberg University, 68167 Mannheim, Germany
4 Department of Anesthesiology and Intensive Care Medicine, Ludwigshafen Hospital, 67063 Ludwigshafen, Germany
5 Department of Anesthesiology and Intensive Care Medicine, University Hospital Ulm, 89081 Ulm, Germany
6 Department of Cranio-Maxillo-Facial-Surgery, Ludwigshafen Hospital, 67063 Ludwigshafen, Germany
* Correspondence: ansakkas@yahoo.de; Tel.: +49-731-1710-1728

Abstract: The primary aim of this study was to assess the incidence of a difficult airway and emergency tracheostomy in patients with orofacial infections originating in the mandible, and a secondary aim was to determine the potential predictors of difficult intubation. This retrospective single-center study included all patients who were referred between 2015 and 2022 with an orofacial infection originating in the mandible and who were surgically drained under intubation anesthesia. The incidence of a difficult airway regarding ventilation, laryngoscopy, and intubation was analyzed descriptively. Associations between potential influencing factors and difficult intubation were examined via multivariable analysis. A total of 361 patients (mean age: 47.7 years) were included in the analysis. A difficult airway was present in 121/361 (33.5%) patients. Difficult intubation was most common in patients with infections of the massetericomandibular space (42.6%), followed by infections of the mouth floor (40%) and pterygomandibular space (23.5%). Dyspnea and stridor were not associated with the localization of infection ($p = 0.6486/p = 0.4418$). Multivariable analysis revealed increased age, restricted mouth opening, higher Mallampati scores, and higher Cormack–Lehane classification grades as significant predictors of difficult intubation. Higher BMI, dysphagia, dyspnea, stridor and a non-palpable mandibular rim did not influence the airway management. Patients with a difficult airway were more likely to be admitted to the ICU after surgery than patients with regular airway were ($p = 0.0001$). To conclude, the incidence of a difficult airway was high in patients with orofacial infections originating in the mandible. Older age, limited mouth opening, a higher Mallampati score, and a higher Cormack–Lehane grade were reliable predictors of difficult intubation.

Keywords: airway management; tracheostomy; intubation; orofacial infection; odontogenic abscess; mandibular infections

1. Introduction

Odontogenic infections are caused by untreated dental caries, periodontal disease, or trauma and are a common reason for seeking medical care in oral and maxillofacial surgery units [1–3]. Data from developed countries suggest that the rate and severity of odontogenic infections in patients who present to hospital emergency departments are increasing [4,5]. Immediate surgical incision and drainage combined with intravenous administration of antibiotics remains the standard treatment [6,7].

If the primary cause of orofacial infections in the mandible spaces is not promptly eliminated, swelling into the cervical multilayered deep fascia can occur, leading to infection in the deep neck space [8]. The severity of these infections can be decreased via surgical clearance and antibiotics, but if the infection spreads, it can obstruct the airway, leading to morbidity and, in rare cases, mortality [8–11]. Extended orofacial infections are challenging because of the complex anatomy of the head and neck, the vicinity of vital structures, and the risk of the infection spreading to adjacent spaces. The location of the infection can also affect airway management, and concomitant trismus can hinder conventional laryngoscopy and intubation [11,12]. The risk of airway compromise is particularly high in patients with infections in several musculofascial spaces [6].

Airway management in patients with abscesses in the perimandibular space is challenging because of swelling, restricted mouth opening, and neck stiffness. Further risk factors for anesthesia-related complications include stridor, neck operations, dysgnathia, restricted head reclination, a reduced thyreomental distance, sleep apnea syndrome, and Mallampati grade III or IV, and these factors have to be considered carefully [13]. Appropriate preoperative assessment and a safe airway are the hallmarks for successful treatment and fewer morbidity-related complications [14]. Modern airway management, including video laryngoscope and fiberoptic methods, can achieve successful intubation even in challenging cases. However, the specific demographic and clinical features that indicate a difficult airway need to be recognized early on. Accurate prediction of a difficult airway has also been associated with successful intubation on the first attempt [15].

Faster and safer surgical treatment reduces the inpatient hospital stay and thereby the economic burden on the healthcare system. Thus, a multidisciplinary approach involving oral and maxillofacial surgeons, anesthesiologists, and emergency medicine physicians is essential for a successful outcome. Although the clinical presentation and treatment outcomes of odontogenic infections have been well reported, the airway management of patients with extended infections originating in the mandible has not been well studied [1,2,4,16]. Since exploration and advancement in personalized medicine is a rapidly growing domain nowadays, distinguishing the airway management of an individual with mandible-related orofacial infection from others with similar clinical presentations can improve diagnosis, reduce complications, and develop outcomes [17].

The primary aim of this study was to assess the incidence of a difficult airway and emergency tracheostomy in patients with orofacial infections originating in the mandible, and a secondary aim was to determine potential predictors of difficult intubation. The length of hospitalization, incidence of surgical revisions, and rate of in-hospital mortality were also evaluated retrospectively.

2. Materials and Methods

For this observational retrospective single-center study, we reviewed the medical records of all patients with orofacial infections/abscesses originating in the mandible who were surgically treated under general anesthesia in our department of oral and plastic maxillofacial surgery between January 2015 and August 2022. Records were retrieved from our hospital electronic database. Ethical approval for this study was obtained from the ethics committee of the chamber of physicians in Rhineland-Palatine, Mainz, Germany (approval number: 2022-16439, approval date: 8 April 2022), and the study was performed in accordance with the Declaration of Helsinki 1964 and its later amendments (World Medical Association, Declaration of Helsinki).

We enrolled patients with an orofacial infection/abscess in the perimandibular spaces that originated in the mandible and who underwent surgical drainage through a cervical approach under intubation anesthesia. Patients were excluded if the orofacial infection did not involve the mandible or adjacent areas, if they underwent surgical drainage under local anesthesia, if no surgical intervention was performed, or if their medical charts were incomplete.

2.1. Patient Screening

Our standard clinical protocol included clinical assessment, laboratory tests, and an initial computer tomography (CT) scan. Patients with swelling around the mandibular area were clinically evaluated for dysphagia, dyspnea, stridor, the palpability of the caudal mandibular rim, and mouth opening. Any clinical information not in the emergency department report was assumed as negative. Extraoral surgical drainage under general anesthesia was indicated by a board-certified oral and maxillofacial surgeon after the evaluation of the clinical and radiological findings. No cases of intraoral drainage were documented.

Extraoral surgical drainage was performed with a submandibular incision in the cervical skin fold, two finger widths below the mandibular rim to protect the marginal branch of the facial nerve, in the direction of the nerve. After blunt preparation of the mandibular rim using blunt dissecting scissors, the lingual and vestibular/submental margins were exposed under constant bone contact. After pus was discharged, a microbiological smear was taken and the wound cavity was irrigated with a disinfecting agent. Two drainage tubes were inserted with grain forceps and fixed with skin sutures. The cause of the infection was also eliminated. All patients received intravenously administered antibiotics from the time of admission until home discharge.

The removal of the intraoral source of infection was addressed in the same or secondary operation, depending on the specific cause and its extension. In cases of odontogenic focus caused by chronic apical parodontitis, the infected teeth were extracted always simultaneously to the extraoral surgical drainage. Tooth extractions were performed only under intubation anesthesia. When the infective cause was an ARONJ or osteomyelitis, sequestrectomy and bone decortication were performed secondarily in the same or a further in-patient hospital stay. Orofacial abscesses following osteotomies, dental implantations or osteosynthesis were treated only with extraoral surgical drainage, mostly under intubation anesthesia but also with a laryngeal mask when possible.

A difficult airway was defined by the presence of difficult ventilation, difficult laryngoscopy, or difficult intubation, according to the current German guidelines [13]. A difficult airway was defined after traditional mask ventilation and intubation using direct laryngoscopy was attempted by a board-certificated anesthetist. Ventilation using the face mask or an extraglottic airway device was defined as difficult or impossible if ventilation was insufficient or completely unsuccessful because of leakage or/and resistance during inspiration or expiration. Ventilation was also defined as difficult if several attempts were needed to place the extraglottic airway device. Difficult laryngoscopy was defined as Cormack–Lehane grade of III or IV and was identified via direct laryngoscopy [18]. The laryngoscopic view was assessed and graded according to the final intubation attempt after each intubation was finished. Difficult endotracheal intubation was defined by the need for several intubation attempts.

Emergency tracheotomy was performed in an awake setting in patients with a clearly compromised airway, who could either be sufficiently ventilated or intubated preoperatively. A secondary tracheotomy was performed during the post-operative stay at the intensive care unit (ICU) electively in patients with resistant soft tissue swelling and high infection parameters, who required prolonged intubation. All tracheotomized patients were decanulated according to regressed soft tissue swelling and normal respiratory condition, and the tracheostoma was primarily surgically closed before discharge. Primary tracheotomized patients and patients with a difficult airway, concomitant comorbidities and extended orofacial infection who required advanced respiratory support were admitted at the ICU post-operatively for further respiratory monitoring and surveillance. Patients who were admitted at the surgical ward post-operatively were closely monitored by the nursing staff via continuous control of the oxygen saturation and respiratory condition including supporting oxygen administration if needed. The attended oral and maxillofacial surgeon also re-evaluated the patient closely to ensure a safe post-operative course. In case of a respiratory emergency (e.g., desaturation, shallow respiration and shortness of breath), the anesthesiologic team was promptly informed.

2.2. Data Collection

Data were collected from patients' electronic hospital charts and patients were anonymized before data analysis. Extracted data comprised patient age, patient gender, antithrombotic medication, body mass index (BMI), the localization of the infection, clinical symptoms at admission (dysphagia, dyspnea, and stridor), relevant clinical findings (palpability of the mandibular rim and extension of mouth opening), etiology of the abscess, ASA grade, Mallampati score, Cormack–Lehane grade, airway management (difficult/regular), the ventilation method, laryngoscopy and intubation (difficult/regular), and the outcome (admission to the ICU, length of hospitalization, rate of surgical revision, or in-hospital mortality) [18,19]. The Mallampati score or Cormack–Lehane grade could not be ascertained if direct intraoral visualization was not possible because of a restricted mouth opening.

We collected all CT scans prescribed by the attending clinician after the clinical evaluation. To measure interrater reliability, each case was interpreted by two board-certified radiologists. We abstracted all radiological findings that were relevant to abscess formation in the spaces around the mandible (paramandibular, submandibular, perimandibular, mouth floor, submental, massetericomandibular, pterygomandibular, and parapharyngeal space). The exact diagnosis and localization of the infection were determined from the operation and radiological report.

2.3. Statistical Analysis

Data were centralized in an electronic format using Microsoft Excel software and analyzed descriptively. Statistical analysis was performed using SAS®, Release 9.4 software (SAS Institute Inc., Cary, NC, USA). Descriptive statistics were used to describe baseline patient characteristics. All categorical variables were expressed as absolute values (n) and relative incidences (%). For metric variables, the standard deviation was calculated. A multivariable analysis was performed to find associations between the possible influencing variables and a difficult airway. Associations between categorical variables were described with cross-tabulations, and chi-square tests were used to investigate a potential association between infection localization, clinical features and a difficult airway. Fisher's exact test was used to compare smaller subgroups. The Cochran–Armitage trend test was used to detect associations between age, BMI, Mallampati score, Cormack–Lehane grade, and the intubation modality. A t-test was used to compare the length of hospital stay in tracheotomized and non-tracheotomized patients. A two-sided p value of less than 0.05 was considered statistically significant.

3. Results

3.1. Demographic Distribution

A total of 361 patients were included in the analysis. There were more males (196/361; 54.3%) than females (165/361; 45.7%) and the male:female ratio was 1.18:1. The patients' age at the time of injury was 5–92 years, and the mean ± SD age was 47.75 ± 19.57 years. Most patients (46.8%) were older than 50 years. The mean ± SD BMI at the time of admission was 26.8 ± 6.59. The baseline patient characteristics are presented in Table 1.

Table 1. Baseline demographics, clinical and anesthesiologic findings and outcome of the overall study population.

		Study Population	
		n	%
Total		361	100.0%
Gender			
	male	196	54.3%
	female	165	45.7%

Table 1. *Cont.*

	Study Population	
	n	%
Age		
<30 years	79	21.9%
≤30–50 years	113	31.3%
≥50 years	169	46.8%
BMI		
<24.9	160	44.3%
≤25–29.9	106	29.4%
≥30	95	26.3%
ASA		
1	87	24.1%
2	218	60.4%
3	55	15.2%
4	1	0.3%
Infection localization		
paramandibular	3	0.8%
submandibular	111	30.7%
perimandibular	168	46.5%
mouth floor	5	1.4%
Submental	36	10.0%
Massetericomandibular	7	1.9%
pterygomandibular	17	4.7%
parapharyngeal	14	3.9%
Infection etiology		
chronic apical parodontitis	270	74.8%
Antiresorptiv-related osteonecrosis of the jaw	7	1.9%
osteomyelitis	6	1.7%
post-osteotomy	60	16.6%
post-implantation	7	1.9%
post-osteosynthesis	2	0.6%
sialadenitis from submandibular gland	2	0.6%
Unknown	7	1.9%
Clinical symptoms		
dysphagia	330	91.4%
dyspnea	12	3.3%
stridor	4	1.1%
Clinical findings		
mandibular rim non-palpable	295	81.7%
restricted mouth opening	348	96.4%

Table 1. *Cont.*

	Study Population	
	n	%
Mallampati score		
1	29	8.0%
2	98	27.1%
3	59	16.3%
4	42	11.6%
5	1	0.3%
No ascertainable	132	36.6%
Cormack–Lehane grade		
1	167	46.3%
2	91	25.2%
3	57	15.8%
4	12	3.3%
No ascertainable	34	9.4%
Admission disposition		
surgical ward	345	95.6%
ICU	16	4.4%
surgical revision	22	6.1%
Death	1	0.3%

Abbreviations: n = number; % = percentage; BMI = body mass index; ASA = American Society of Anesthesiology.

3.2. Etiology and Localization of Infection

The most common etiology of infection was chronic apical periodontitis (n = 270; 74.8%), followed by infections post-osteotomy (n = 60; 16.6%). Infections were most common in the perimandibular space (n = 168; 46.5%), followed by the submandibular space (n = 111; 30.7%) and the submental space (n = 36; 10%) (Table 1). Dysphagia was detected significantly more often in patients with submental infections (Fischer's exact test: $p = 0.0065$), while a non-palpable mandibular rim was documented significantly more often in patients with infections of the submandibular space (Chi-square test: $p < 0.0001$), perimandibular space (Chi-square test: $p < 0.0001$), mouth floor (Fischer's exact test: $p = 0.0002$), submental area (Chi-square test: $p = 0.0373$), and parapharyngeal area (Fischer's exact test: $p < 0.0001$). Dyspnea and stridor were not associated with the localization of infection (Fischer's exact test: $p = 0.6486$ and $p = 0.4418$, respectively).

3.3. Airway Management

Cervical surgical drainage was performed within the first 24 h after admission in all patients.

Ventilation was defined as difficult in 10.2% (n = 37/361) of patients and an extraglottic airway device was used. Laryngoscopy was difficult in 28.5% (n = 103/361) of patients and intubation was difficult in 19.9% (n = 72/361) of patients. A difficult airway was documented in 121 (33.5%) patients (Figure 1).

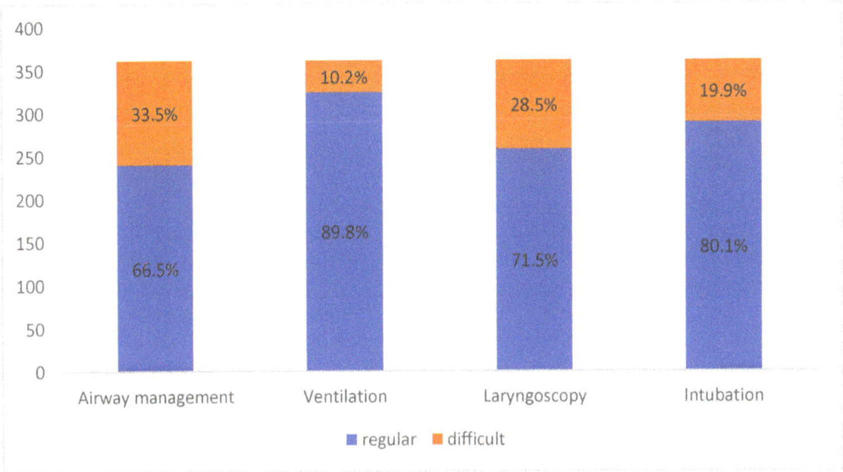

Figure 1. Airway modality regarding ventilation, laryngoscopy and intubation according to the study's definition criteria of a difficult airway.

One hundred and ten patients (30.5%) underwent nasotracheal intubation, 243 patients (67.3%) underwent orotracheal intubation and seven patients (1.9%) were fitted with a laryngeal mask. One patient (0.3%) with a paraphyryngeal abscess was primarily tracheotomized in an awake setting by a "cannot intubate, cannot ventilate" situation. In patients anesthetized with a laryngeal mask, only extraoral surgical drainage was performed without intraoral intervention. Rapid-sequence induction was performed in seven patients (1.9%) because of extensive swelling and progressive dyspnea. Intubation was laryngoscopic in 295 patients (81.7%), bronchoscopic in 17 patients (4.7%), and awake-fiberoptic in 41 patients (11.4%) (Figure 2).

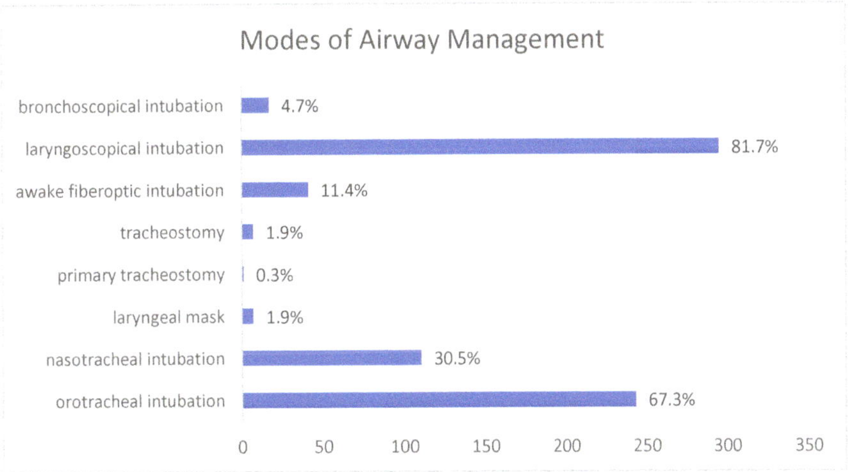

Figure 2. Different modes of airway management in the study population.

Of the patients, 345 (95.5%) were extubated immediately after surgery and 16 patients (4.5%) remained intubated and were admitted to the ICU for further observation. Secondary tracheotomy was performed in six (1.6%) patients during the ICU stay because of resistant swelling and the need for prolonged intubation.

Of 121 patients with a difficult airway, 10.5% (n = 13) required post-operative monitoring in the ICU and 89.5% (n = 108) were transferred to the normal surgical ward. Only 1.2% of patients with regular airway management (n = 3/240) needed intensive care, and 98.8% (n = 237/240) were transferred to the normal surgical ward (chi-square test: p = 0.0001).

3.4. Multivariable Analysis

The multivariable analysis revealed older age, restricted mouth opening, higher Mallampati scores, and higher Cormack–Lehane classification grades as significant predictors of difficult intubation.

Difficult intubation was documented in 5/79 (6.3%) patients younger than 30 years of age, in 22/113 (19.4%) patients aged between 30 and 50 years, and in 45/169 (26.6%) patients older than 50 years. Increasing age significantly increased the risk of difficult intubation (Cochran–Armitage trend test: p = 0.0002). Difficult intubation was detected in 17.5% (28/160) of patients with a BMI of < 24.9, in 19.8% (21/106) of patients with a BMI of 25–29.9, and in 24.2% (23/95) of patients with a BMI of $\geq$ 30 (Cochran–Armitage trend test: p = 0.2013).

Difficult intubation was most common in patients with infections of the massetericomandibular space (42.6%), followed by patients with infections of the mouth floor (40%) and pterygomandibular space (23.5%), but these differences were not significant (p > 0.05) (Table 2).

Table 2. Correlation between infection localization and intubation modality.

Infection Localization	Intubation					
	Difficult		Regular		Total	p Value
	n/%		n/%			
paramandibular	0	0%	3	100%	3	** 1.000
submandibular	19	17.1%	92	82.9%	111	* 0.3703
perimandibular	35	20.8%	133	79.2%	168	* 0.6934
mouth floor	2	40.0%	3	60%	5	** 0.2610
submental	7	19.4%	29	80.6%	36	* 0.9369
massetericomandibular	3	42.6%	4	57.4%	7	** 0.1451
pterygomandibular	4	23.5%	13	76.5%	17	** 0.7554
parapharyngeal	2	14.2%	12	85.8%	14	** 0.7449
Total	72	19.9%	289	80.1%	361	

Abbreviations: n = number; % = percentage; significance level = 0.05. * Chi-square test. ** Fischer's exact test.

We also examined the correlation between patient's symptoms at the initial examination and the occurrence of difficult intubation (Table 3). Of the patients, 25% (n = 3/12) with dysphagia and 25% (n = 3/12) with dyspnea experienced a difficult intubation. A difficult intubation was also observed in two out of four (50%) patients with initial stridor. Difficult intubation occurred in 21% (62/295) of the patients in whom the mandibular rim could not be consistently palpated during clinical examination and in 15.2% (n = 10/66) of patients with a consistently palpable mandibular rim. Difficult intubation was detected in 18.9% of patients with a restricted mouth opening (n = 66/348). Only a restricted mouth opening was significantly associated with an increased rate of difficult intubation.

Table 3. Correlation between infection-relevant clinical symptoms/findings and intubation modality.

Clinical Symptoms/Findings		Intubation					
		Difficult		Regular		Total	p Value
		n/%		n/%			
dysphagia	yes	3	25%	9	75%	12	** 0.7123
	no	69	19.8%	280	80.2%	349	
dyspnea	yes	3	25%	9	75%	12	** 0.7123
	no	69	19.8%	280	80.2%	349	
stridor	yes	2	50%	2	50%	4	** 0.1791
	no	70	19.6%	287	80.4%	357	
mandibular rim	not palpable	62	21.%	233	79%	295	* 0.2810
	palpable	10	15.2%	56	84.8%	66	
restricted mouth opening	yes	66	18.9%	272	81.1%	348	** 0.031
	no	6	46.1%	7	53.9%	13	
Total		72	19.9%	289	80.1%	361	

Abbreviations: n = number; % = percentage; significance level = 0.05. * Chi-square test. ** Fischer's exact test.

Higher Mallampati scores and Cormack–Lehane classifications were significantly associated with an increased risk of difficult intubation (Cochran–Armitage trend test: $p < 0.0001$) (Table 4).

Table 4. Correlation between Mallampati and Cormack–Lehane classification grade and intubation modality.

Mallampati Score	Intubation					
	Difficult		Regular		Total	p Value
	n/%		n/%			
1	1	3.5%	28	96.5%	29	* < 0.0001
2	10	10.2%	88	89.8%	98	
3	12	20.3%	47	79.7%	59	
4	20	47.65	22	52.4%	42	
5	1	100%	0	0%	1	
No ascertainable	28	21.2%	104	78.8%	132	
Total	72	19.9%	289	80.1%	361	
Cormack–Lehane grade	Intubation					
	difficult		regular		Total	p value
	n/%		n/%			
1	5	3%	162	97%	167	* < 0.0001
2	7	7.7%	84	92.3%	91	
3	27	47.4%	30	52.6%	57	
4	11	91.7%	1	8.3%	12	
No ascertainable	22	64.7%	12	35.3%	34	
Total	72		289		361	

Abbreviations: n = number; % = percentage; significance level = 0.05. * Cochran–Armitage trend test.

3.5. Post-operative Outcome

The mean post-operative length of hospitalization was 6.08 days (range: 1–66 days). The length of stay was significantly shorter for patients without a tracheostomy (mean: 5.5 days; range: 1–20 days) than for tracheotomized patients (mean: 35.4 days; range: 9–66 days) (t-test: $p = 0.0194$) (Figure 3).

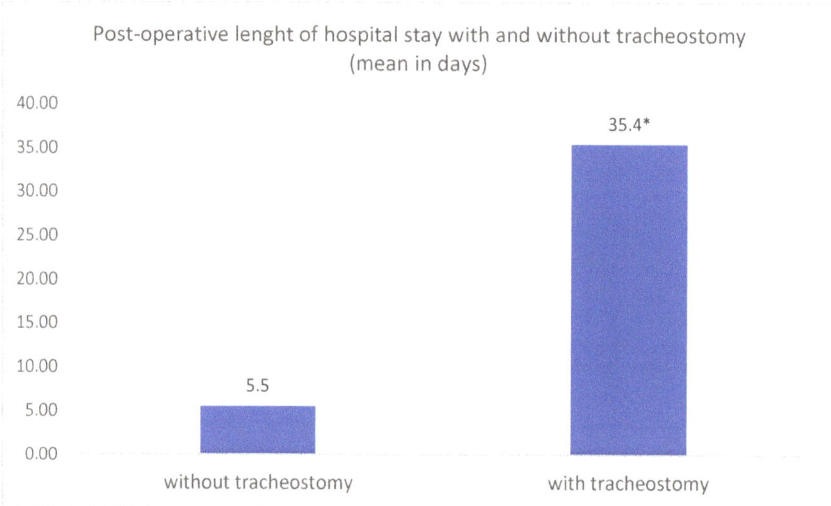

Figure 3. Comparative analysis of mean post-operative length of hospital stay in patients with and without tracheostomy. * t-test: $p = 0.0194$.

Of the 121 patients with a difficult airway, 10.5% required monitoring in the ICU and 89.5% were transferred to the normal surgical ward after surgery. Only 1.2% of patients with regular airway management required intensive care; the remaining 98.8% ($n = 237/240$) were transferred to the normal surgical ward (Fischer's exact test: $p < 0.0001$). In total, 11 out of 72 patients (15.3%) with a difficult intubation and 5 out of 189 patients (1.7%) with a regular intubation were admitted post-operatively to the ICU for further observation (Fischer's exact test: $p < 0.0001$). The 16 intubated patients were treated in the ICU for a mean period of 6.6 days (range: 1–23 days). Seven of the tracheotomized patients stayed for a mean period of 11.7 days (range: 1–23 days) and nine of the patients without tracheostomy stayed for a mean period of 2.7 days (range: 1–5 days).

The in-hospital mortality rate was 0.3% ($n = 1/361$). A 56-year-old male with a parapharyngeal infection of unknown origin who initially presented with dysphagia, dyspnea, and stridor died 3 days post-operatively after developing cardiogenic shock. Twenty-two patients (6.1%) underwent surgical re-drainage during hospitalization because of persistent swelling and elevated laboratory infection parameters.

4. Discussion

We aimed to specify the clinical features that predict a difficult airway and difficult intubation in patients with orofacial infections originating in the mandible. Our results provide valuable insights into how preoperative evaluation of these patients can increase the safety of airway management during surgical treatment of orofacial infections. Considering the challenges and features of personalized medicine and dentistry nowadays, through this article we aimed to apply our collective knowledge with regard to precise risk factors to enable an individualized therapy and develop precision health care [17].

Most reported orofacial infections have an odontogenic cause, and chronic apical periodontitis was the most common cause of infection in our study [1–4]. This is in agreement with the findings of Tapiovaara and Kinzer et al., who found that odontogenic infections can lead to necrotizing fasciitis with a mediastinal extension [11,20]. Postsurgical infection (such as after osteotomies, dental implantations, or trauma surgery) was the next most common cause of infection in our cohort, followed by antiresorptiva-related osteonecrosis of the jaw. These findings show a high possibility of severe infection after oral surgery; therefore, we recommend intensive post-operative care and evaluation to avoid this, especially in immunosuppressed patients.

The affected anatomic space is important for the surgical and anesthesiologic treatment of an infection. In our study, more than 75% of infections were detected in the perimandibular and submandibular space. These spaces are likely commonly affected by infection because of their close anatomic relationship with the roots of the posterior mandibular molars [1]. However, contrary to our initial hypothesis, the localization of infection was not correlated with an increased risk of difficult intubation. We agree with Bowe et al., that trismus is more severe when more spaces are involved [1]. Infection of the masticatory muscles can reduce mouth opening, thereby restricting intraoral access for anesthesiologic management. In these cases, fiberoptic intubation and an experienced consultant anesthetist is needed. In our study, 11.4% of the patients needed awake fiberoptic intubation. This was decided for patients with extended abscesses and combined trismus, who had a history of a difficult airway after previous operations or with a clear risk of an impossible direct laryngoscopy determined in advance. We encourage awake fiberoptic intubation in high-risk patients because intubation can be performed prior to the induction of general anesthesia with its possible risks of inadequate oxygenation, loss of upper airway consistency, and failed intubation. However, an adequate time for preparation and a cooperative patient are required for a safe and successful procedure. We agree with Bowe et al., that using CT scans to monitor orofacial infections is a valuable way to indicate potential airway compromise [1]. Based on these observations, we recommend close preoperative communication between anesthesiologists and surgeons to guarantee the best post-operative outcome, especially in cases of perimandibular and submandibular abscesses.

Surgical drainage of abscesses in the lower orofacial spaces is a short procedure, and the airway tract is often edematous, which increases the risk of airway compromise [14]. Careful preoperative assessment is crucial in these patients to select the appropriate airway modality. Clinical features for assessing airway difficulty include the mouth opening, the Mallampati score, palpability of the mandibular rim, and symptoms such as dysphagia, dyspnea, and stridor. All patients in this study were referred with definitive infection-related swelling that required surgical drainage. Cervical access was necessary for drainage because the extended trismus prevented intraoral access.

In our study, most intubations were laryngoscopic and 33.5% of patients had a compromised airway. These findings cannot be compared with those of other studies because the published definitions of a difficult airway vary widely [13]. Problems during endotracheal intubation are often referred to as "difficult intubation" without distinguishing between "laryngoscopy" and "intubation". These terms need to be separated because anatomical and optical axes converge in laryngoscopy and an acceptable laryngoscopic result can lead to a successful intubation. The rate of difficult ventilation was 10.2% in our study, which is higher than the rates published in other studies [13,21,22]. We also reported a higher rate of difficult direct laryngoscopy (28.5%) than did other studies (1.5–13.45%) [13,23,24]. However, our findings cannot be directly compared with those of other studies because of differences in protocol and patient sample.

We performed surgery under laryngeal mask airway in only seven cases. These patients received extraoral drainage of abscesses following dental implantations or dentoalveolar procedures without further intraoral intervention. The use of a laryngeal mask can be useful in emergency cases of difficult or impossible intubation, when the patient appears to be in stable condition, and the duration of the planned surgical procedure is quite short. However, this airway management method does not support intraoral interventions and should not be preferred when the intraoral infective source has to be removed simultaneously.

We had one unexpected "cannot intubate, cannot ventilate" situation in our cohort, in a patient with a paraphyryngeal abscess [13,23]. This patient received a primary tracheostomy. This is similar to the findings of Motahari et al. and Kataria et al., who reported peritonsillar abscesses requiring primary tracheostomy in 1% and 5% of patients [25,26]. We did not observe enough tracheostomy cases to determine the correlation between the localization of infection and rate of tracheostomy. In our cohort, 6/16 patients who were admitted to the ICU were tracheotomized because of persistent swelling and prolonged intubation. We agree with Tapiovaara et al., that tracheostomy can avoid laryngeal injury in patients needing prolonged intubation, thereby reducing the need for sedation and mechanical ventilation [11]. Early tracheostomy has been correlated with lower mortality rates in patients with deep neck infections [27]. However, we believe that tracheostomy can be avoided by proper preoperative airway planning. If emergency intubation is needed, for example in more challenging patients, we recommend securing the patient's airway via awake intubation and video laryngoscopy under sedation by experienced anesthesiologists.

We identified four predictors of difficult intubation: older age, limited mouth opening, a higher Mallampati score, and a higher Cormack–Lehane grade. These predictors may be able to be used to identify patients with difficult intubation following either conventional direct laryngoscopy or indirect laryngoscopy with fiberoptic methods. These factors can also be used to identify patients at risk of a difficult airway in the preoperative anesthesiologic assessment. Unexpectedly, a higher BMI was not associated with an increased rate of difficult intubation. Similarly, dysphagia, dyspnea, stridor and a non-palpable mandibular rim as clinical symptoms of a difficult airway that could be assumed in advance were also not correlated to higher risk for difficult intubation. Further studies are needed to develop an intubation prediction score for determining the risk of difficult intubation in patients with orofacial infections.

We found that difficult intubation was more common in patients older than 50 years than in younger patients. This finding is consistent with that of previous studies that have shown an association between increased age and difficult airway management [21,22,24]. The increased risk of a difficult airway in older individuals could be due to age-related changes in the airway anatomy of these individuals, such as decreased elasticity, decreased muscle tone, and decreased neck mobility. The increased risk of difficult intubation in older individuals may be due to the anterior shift of the mandible relative to the maxilla caused by the attrition of the molar cusps and the regeneration of the cementum [28]. Intubation difficulties may also be caused by age-related disc displacement and osteoarthritis of the temporomandibular joint, which can restrict mouth opening, as well as by mandibular resorption and alveolar remodeling, which can cause jaw retraction and drooping, making mask ventilation and laryngoscopy more difficult [28]. Kyphotic deformities and poor neck mobility may also contribute to this problem [21,22,24]. In addition, fibroblast proliferation decreased with age, which reduces the flexibility and elasticity of the oral cavity, thereby limiting mouth opening. This may also contribute to difficult airway management in older individuals [29].

The risk of difficult intubation was higher in patients with a BMI of ≥ 30. These findings are consistent with those of previous studies [30,31]. Difficult airway management in obese patients may be caused by the larger neck circumference, increased fat deposition in the upper airway, and decreased lung volume in these individuals. We also observed a significantly higher rate of difficult intubation in underweight patients in out cohort, likely due to the smaller dimensions of the lower face.

Surprisingly, we found no correlation between the localization of the infection and modality of the intubation. We expected patients with abscesses in the mouth floor, pterygomandibular space, or parapharyngeal space to have a more demanding airway because of tissue edema, an obstructed upper airway, and jaw immobility, but this was not confirmed—possibly because we only had a few patients with these infections in our cohort. As expected, patients with paramandibular and submental abscesses had the lowest risk of having a difficult airway, likely because these spaces are anatomically more distant from the respiratory tract and mouth-opening muscles.

The incidence of difficult intubation was higher in patients with higher Mallampati scores and Cormack–Lehane grades, which is in accordance with published findings [13]. We did not find any association between clinical symptoms (such as dysphagia, dyspnea, and stridor) and intubation modality, possibly because of the small number of patients with these symptoms. Only limited mouth opening was associated with increased intubation difficulty, which has been confirmed in past studies [13,24]. However, we recommend examining patients carefully for these symptoms as they may predict difficult or impossible direct laryngoscopy or intubation.

As expected, difficult airway management was a significant risk factor for ICU admission after surgery. In our cohort, the rate of post-operative admission to the ICU was 4.4% and the mean ICU stay length was 6.6 days. This was higher than the ICU admission rate of 0.4% and longer than the mean ICU stay length of 4 days reported by Bowe [1]. Tapiovaara et al. reported a longer median ICU stay of 7 days [11]. Case numbers were too low to detect a correlation between the localization of infection and the duration of ICU stay.

Patients who underwent tracheostomy had a significantly longer hospital stay than did patients who did not undergo tracheostomy. This can be explained by the significantly advanced disease that necessitates tracheostomy in the first place [11,32,33]. In support of our findings, Nagarkar et al. also found a significantly longer hospital stay following tracheostomy, but this was following head and neck cancer surgeries [14].

Delaying surgical treatment of orofacial infections can make anesthesiologic treatment more challenging and increase the overall duration of hospital stay. Coexisting medical conditions can also increase the risk of severe infection or sepsis. Most studies recommend the immediate surgical drainage of abscesses combined with the intravenous administration of antibiotics in odontogenic or deep neck infections; however, the optimal timing of surgery is still under debate [2,7,34,35]. All patients in this cohort were operated on within the first day of admission. In concordance with others, we strongly recommend early surgical drainage and the simultaneous intravenous administration of antibiotics to avoid compromising the airway further [36,37].

There are some limitations to this study. First, the study was restricted to one emergency care unit so the results may not be generalizable to other centers. Second, the retrospective nature of the research may have caused documentation bias; however, this limitation was outweighed by the large study cohort. Third, the different level of education and experience of the treating physicians in our study may have biased our results. Data were collected from medical records completed by the intubator, which could have caused observer bias with regard to the intubation approach. As a result, the choice of airway management and its difficulty could only be evaluated subjectively. Fourth, several evidence-based clinical predictors of a difficult airway, such as previous operations, radiation of the head/neck area, sleep apnea syndrome, mandibular protrusion, thyreomental distance, and macroglossia could not be extracted from the patients' files. Fifth, we did not compare our patient sample with a control cohort of patients with orofacial infections originating in the maxilla or other anatomic spaces, so our findings are limited to infections in the mandible. Sixth, we included patients of all ages, so our results cannot be generalized to a specific age group. Finally, we did not evaluate the influence of the microbiological examination of pus swabs and of systemic health on the duration of hospitalization in our study. This could have introduced a bias to our findings since the length of stay does not depend only on airway management [38]. Future prospective studies with standardized protocols are warranted to validate our preliminary findings.

5. Conclusions

The incidence of a difficult airway was 33.5% in our cohort of patients with orofacial infections originating in the mandible. Factors increasing the risk of a difficult intubation were older age, limited mouth opening, higher Mallampati scores, and higher Cormack–Lehane grades. We recommend the careful evaluation of these factors preoperatively as a way of reliably predicting difficult intubation. Difficult intubation was most common in patients with infections of the massetericomandibular space, followed by infections of the mouth floor and pterygomandibular space, albeit without statistical significance. A higher BMI, dysphagia, dyspnea, stridor and a non-palpable mandibular rim did not influence airway management. We highlight the importance of clear communication between surgeons and anesthesiologists to determine the safest airway approach during surgery. Fiberoptic orotracheal intubation is the most appropriate technique for managing a difficult airway in patients with these orofacial infections. Although tracheostomy is both rare and safe, individual assessment and proper preoperative planning is required. The modalities of airway management and tracheostomy have a significant impact on the post-operative length of hospital stay. These findings will help clinicians to reduce the risk of complications and improve patient safety during airway management. Our preliminary results and recommendations should be confirmed by well-designed prospective studies.

Author Contributions: Conceptualization, A.S.; Methodology, A.S., M.S., S.P., F.W. and M.E.; Software, C.W.; Investigation, A.S. and C.A.R.; Resources, A.S.; Data curation, C.W.; Writing—original draft, A.S.; Writing—review & editing, O.C.T. and M.E.; Visualization, O.C.T. and M.E.; Supervision, W.Z. and R.A.M.; Project administration, R.A.M. All authors have read and agreed to the published version of the manuscript.

Funding: This research received no external funding.

Institutional Review Board Statement: Ethical approval for this study was obtained from the ethics committee of the chamber of physicians in Rhineland-Palatine, Mainz, Germany (approval number: 2022-16439, approval date: 8 April 2022). This research was conducted in full accordance with the ethical standards of the institutional research committee as well as with the 1964 Helsinki declaration and its later amendments or comparable ethical standards. For this non-interventional observational retrospective study, all data were also anonymized and de-identified prior to analysis and no written consent of the patient was obtained. Full compliance with data protection and safeguarding of data were ensured and no information which could identify the patients was collected. Reporting was based on the recommendations of the Strengthening the Reporting of Observational Studies in Epidemiology (STROBE) initiative [39].

Informed Consent Statement: Not applicable.

Data Availability Statement: The datasets generated and analyzed during the current study are not publicly available due to institutional restrictions, but are available from the corresponding author upon reasonable request.

Acknowledgments: The authors like to thank Dr. Claire Bacon for the language editing of this manuscript.

Conflicts of Interest: The authors declare that they have no competing or financial interests, either directly or indirectly, in the products listed in the study. This research did not receive any specific grant from funding agencies in the public, commercial, or not-for-profit sectors.

References

1. Bowe, C.M.; O'Neill, M.A.; O'Connell, J.E.; Kearns, G.J. The surgical management of severe dentofacial infections (DFI)-a prospective study. *Ir. J. Med. Sci.* **2019**, *188*, 327–331. [CrossRef]
2. Cambria, F.; Fusconi, M.; Candelori, F.; Galli, M.; Stanganelli, F.R.F.; Venuta, F.; Valentini, V.; de Vincentiis, M. Surgical multidisciplinary approach in the management of odontogenic or non-odontogenic neck infections. *Acta Otorhinolaryngol. Ital.* **2021**, *41*, 138–144. [CrossRef]
3. Buckley, J.; Harris, A.S.; Addams-Williams, J. Ten years of deep neck space abscesses. *J. Laryngol. Otol.* **2019**, *133*, 324–328. [CrossRef]
4. Fu, B.; McGowan, K.; Sun, J.H.; Batstone, M. Increasing frequency and severity of odontogenic infection requiring hospital admission and surgical management. *Br. J. Oral. Maxillofac. Surg.* **2020**, *58*, 409–415. [CrossRef]

5. Salomon, D.; Heidel, R.E.; Kolokythas, A.; Miloro, M.; Schlieve, T. Does restriction of public health care dental benefits affect the volume, severity, or cost of dental related hospital visits? *J. Oral. Maxillofac. Surg.* **2017**, *75*, 467–474. [CrossRef]
6. Mücke, T.; Dujka, N.; Ermer, M.A.; Wolff, K.D.; Kesting, M.; Mitchell, D.A.; Ritschl, L.; Deppe, H. The value of early intraoral incisions in patients with perimandibular odontogenic maxillofacial abscesses. *J. Craniomaxillofac. Surg.* **2015**, *43*, e220–e223. [CrossRef]
7. Heim, N.; Warwas, F.B.; Wiedemeyer, V.; Wilms, C.T.; Reich, R.H.; Martini, M. The role of immediate versus secondary removal of the odontogenic focus in treatment of deep head and neck space infections. A retrospective analysis of 248 patients. *Clin. Oral. Investig.* **2019**, *23*, 2921–2927. [CrossRef]
8. Bhardwaj, R.; Makkar, S.; Gupta, A.; Khandelwal, K.; Nathan, K.; Basu, C.; Palaniyappan, G. Deep Neck Space Infections: Current Trends and Intricacies of Management? *Indian J. Otolaryngol. Head Neck Surg.* **2022**, *74*, 2344–2349. [CrossRef]
9. Ogle, O.E. Odontogenic Infections. *Dental Clin. N. Am.* **2017**, *61*, 235–252. [CrossRef]
10. Bowe, C.M.; Gargan, M.L.; Kearns, G.J.; Stassen, L. Does altered access to general dental treatment affect the number and complexity of patients presenting to the acute hospital service with severe dentofacial infections? *J. Ir. Dent Assoc.* **2015**, *61*, 196–200.
11. Tapiovaara, L.K.; Aro, K.L.S.; Bäck, L.J.J.; Koskinen, A.I.M. Comparison of intubation and tracheotomy in adult patients with acute epiglottitis or supraglottitis. *Eur. Arch. Otorhinolaryngol.* **2019**, *276*, 3173–3177. [CrossRef] [PubMed]
12. Cho, S.Y.; Woo, J.H.; Kim, Y.J.; Chun, E.H.; Han, J.I.; Kim, D.Y.; Baik, H.J.; Chung, R.K. Airway management in patients with deep neck infections: A retrospective analysis. *Medicine* **2016**, *95*, e4125. [CrossRef] [PubMed]
13. Piepho, T.; Cavus, E.; Noppens, R.; Byhahn, C.; Dörges, V.; Zwissler, B.; Timmermann, A. S1 Leitlinie: Atemwegsmanagement Airwaymanagement. AWMF-Register Nr.: 001/028. Available online: https://register.awmf.org/de/leitlinien/detail/001-028 (accessed on 12 March 2015).
14. Nagarkar, R.; Kokane, G.; Wagh, A.; Kulkarni, N.; Roy, S.; Tandale, R.; Pawar, S. Airway management techniques in head and neck cancer surgeries: A retrospective analysis. *Oral. Maxillofac. Surg.* **2019**, *23*, 311–315. [CrossRef] [PubMed]
15. Kim, C.; Kang, H.G.; Lim, T.H.; Choi, B.Y.; Shin, Y.J.; Choi, H.J. What factors affect the success rate of the first attempt at endotracheal intubation in emergency departments? *Emerg. Med. J.* **2013**, *30*, 888–892. [CrossRef]
16. Bertossi, D.; Barone, A.; Iurlaro, A.; Marconcini, S.; De Santis, D.; Finotti, M.; Procacci, P. Odontogenic Orofacial Infections. *J. Craniofac. Surg.* **2017**, *28*, 197–202. [CrossRef]
17. Reddy, M.S.; Shetty, S.R.; Vannala, V. Embracing Personalized Medicine in Dentistry. *J. Pharm. Bioallied. Sci.* **2019**, *11*, 92–96. [CrossRef]
18. Cormack, R.S.; Lehane, J. Difficult tracheal intubation in obstetrics. *Anaesthesia* **1984**, *39*, 1105–1111. [CrossRef]
19. Mallampati, S.R.; Gatt, S.P.; Gugino, L.D.; Desai, S.P.; Waraksa, B.; Freiberger, D.; Liu, P.L. A clinical sign to predict difficult tracheal intubation: A prospective study. *Can. Anaesth. Soc. J.* **1985**, *32*, 429–434. [CrossRef]
20. Kinzer, S.; Pfeifer, J.; Becker, S.; Ridder, G.J. Severe deep neck space infections and mediastinitis of odontogenic origin: Clinical relevance and implications for diagnosis and treatment. *Acta Otolaryngol.* **2009**, *129*, 62–70. [CrossRef]
21. Kheterpal, S.; Han, R.; Tremper, K.K.; Shanks, A.; Tait, A.R.; O'Reilly, M.; Ludwig, T.A. Incidence and predictors of difficult and impossible mask ventilation. *Anesthesiology* **2006**, *105*, 885–891. [CrossRef]
22. Kheterpal, S.; Healy, D.; Aziz, M.F.; Shanks, A.M.; Freundlich, R.E.; Linton, F.; Martin, L.D.; Linton, J.; Epps, J.L.; Fernandez-Bustamante, A.; et al. Multicenter Perioperative Outcomes Group (MPOG) Perioperative Clinical Research Committee. Incidence, predictors, and outcome of difficult mask ventilation combined with difficult laryngoscopy: A report from the multicenter perioperative outcomes group. *Anesthesiology* **2013**, *119*, 1360–1369. [CrossRef] [PubMed]
23. Lavery, G.G.; McCloskey, B.V. The difficult airway in adult critical care. *Crit. Care Med.* **2008**, *36*, 2163–2173. [CrossRef] [PubMed]
24. Savatmongkorngul, S.; Pitakwong, P.; Sricharoen, P.; Yuksen, C.; Jenpanitpong, C.; Watcharakitpaisan, S. Difficult Laryngoscopy Prediction Score for Intubation in Emergency Departments: A Retrospective Cohort Study. *Open Access Emerg. Med.* **2022**, *29*, 311–322. [CrossRef] [PubMed]
25. Motahari, S.J.; Poormoosa, R.; Nikkhah, M.; Bahari, M.; Shirazy, S.M.; Khavarinejad, F. Treatment and prognosis of deep neck infections. *Indian J. Otolaryngol. Head Neck Surg.* **2015**, *67*, 134–137. [CrossRef] [PubMed]
26. Kataria, G.; Saxena, A.; Bhagat, S.; Singh, B.; Kaur, M.; Kaur, G. Deep neck space infections: A study of 76 cases. *Iran J. Otorhinolaryngol.* **2015**, *27*, 293–299.
27. Celakovsky, P.; Kalfert, D.; Tucek, L.; Mejzlik, J.; Kotulek, M.; Vrbacky, A.; Matousek, P.; Stanikova, L.; Hoskova, T.; Pasz, A. Deep neck infections: Risk factors for mediastinal extension. *Eur. Arch. Otorhinolaryngol.* **2014**, *271*, 1679–1683. [CrossRef]
28. Karkouti, K.; Rose, D.K.; Wigglesworth, D.; Cohen, M.M. Predicting difficult intubation: A multivariable analysis. *Can J. Anaesth.* **2000**, *47*, 730–739. [CrossRef]
29. Rossa, B.; Selle, E. Quantitative changes in the elastic fibers of the human oral mucosa of the hard palate and cheek at various ages. *Zahn. Mund Kieferheilkd Zent.* **1984**, *72*, 217–222.
30. Uribe, A.A.; Zvara, D.A.; Puente, E.G.; Otey, A.J.; Zhang, J.; Bergese, S.D. BMI as a Predictor for Potential Difficult Tracheal Intubation in Males. *Front. Med.* **2015**, *4*, 38. [CrossRef]
31. Wang, T.; Sun, S.; Huang, S. The association of body mass index with difficult tracheal intubation management by direct laryngoscopy: A meta-analysis. *BMC Anesth.* **2018**, *30*, 79. [CrossRef]

32. Siddiqui, A.S.; Dogar, S.A.; Lal, S.; Akhtar, S.; Khan, F.A. Airway management and postoperative length of hospital stay in patients undergoing head and neck cancer surgery. *J. Anaesthesiol. Clin. Pharm.* **2016**, *32*, 49–53. [CrossRef] [PubMed]
33. Cameron, M.; Corner, A.; Diba, A.; Hankins, M. Development of a tracheostomy scoring system to guide airway management after major head and neck surgery. *Int. J. Oral. Maxillofac. Surg.* **2009**, *38*, 846–849. [CrossRef]
34. Böttger, S.; Lautenbacher, K.; Domann, E.; Howaldt, H.P.; Attia, S.; Streckbein, P.; Wilbrand, J.F. Indication for an additional postoperative antibiotic treatment after surgical incision of serious odontogenic abscesses. *J. Craniomaxillofac. Surg.* **2020**, *48*, 229–234. [CrossRef] [PubMed]
35. Cramer, J.D.; Purkey, M.R.; Smith, S.S.; Schroeder, J.W., Jr. The impact of delayed surgical drainage of deep neck abscesses in adult and pediatric populations. *Laryngoscope* **2016**, *126*, 1753–1760. [CrossRef] [PubMed]
36. Doll, C.; Carl, F.; Neumann, K.; Voss, J.O.; Hartwig, S.; Waluga, R.; Heiland, M.; Raguse, J.D. Odontogenic Abscess-Related Emergency Hospital Admissions: A Retrospective Data Analysis of 120 Children and Young People Requiring Surgical Drainage. *Biomed. Res. Int.* **2018**, *26*, 3504727. [CrossRef]
37. Kara, A.; Ozsurekci, Y.; Tekcicek, M.; Karadag Oncel, E.; Cengiz, A.B.; Karahan, S.; Ceyhan, M.; Celik, M.O.; Ozkaya-Parlakay, A. Length of hospital stay and management of facial cellulitis of odontogenic origin in children. *Pediatr. Dent.* **2014**, *36*, 18–22.
38. Penel, N.; Mallet, Y.; Roussel-Delvallez, M.; Lefebvre, J.L.; Yazdanpanah, Y. Factors determining length of the postoperative hospital stay after major head and neck cancer surgery. *Oral. Oncol.* **2008**, *44*, 555–562. [CrossRef]
39. Vandenbroucke, J.P.; von Elm, E.; Altman, D.G.; Gøtzsche, P.C.; Mulrow, C.D.; Pocock, S.J.; Poole, C.; Schlesselman, J.J.; Egger, M. STROBE Initiative. Strengthening the Reporting of Observational Studies in Epidemiology (STROBE): Explanation and elaboration. *Int. J. Surg.* **2014**, *12*, 1500–1524. [CrossRef]